BEAUTY IS THE PERFECT GIFT TO WOMEN

-ASHWINI AHUJA

Ladies generally desire to be praised, valued and respected. When their physical appearance improves, a wonder happens. People love paying attention to beautiful and fit women.

Beautiful women are attracted everywhere. A beautiful and healthy woman is more confident, happy and bubbly.

In fact, beauty serves as the foundation of happiness and health. It is an important evolutionary cue. In physical beauty, it is the skin that is the cause of concern for most ladies.

Skin is one of the largest organs of the body. Care of the skin directly affects the health of the complete body.

"Beauty is the perfect gift to women" is a solution to your concerns. This book is about health, beauty and women. It is an ideal book for ladies who desire to glimpse some wonders in their appearance and social life. It is based on several articles already published in different periodicals.

INDEX

Ashwini Ahuja

Chapter One

Belly fit: A Holistic Fitness Experience

At present, our life is stressful, busy, hard and challenging. If we don't care about ourselves, we won't be ready to take care of others. A time has come when the women should be the best, the strongest and the healthiest to cope with the challenges of modern times. Needless to say that bellyfit- a modern holistic fitness experience is designed to connect you to the deep, primal feminine within. Moreover, it helps you gain strength to sort out modern day stress

Have you heard about bellyfit? It is significantly a new fitness style among women across the world. In India, it has charmed the ladies to a great extent thanks to its unique features.

Bellyfit is quite different from conventional physical exercise, dance or yoga. Indeed, it is a fusion of movements inspired by the science of western fitness to burn calories, relieve stress and get the sweat flowing with fun and delight.

Bellyfit is a blending of style and beauty of cultural dance and the power of spiritual practices with the philosophy of east. Bellyfit connoisseurs opine that it is a low impact fitness style that fuses exercises

The main purpose of the bellyfit is to improve strength and the flexibility of the core muscles especially the muscles that are around the waistline.
Fitness expert Sanjeev Marshal says that bellyfit is actually a low impact fitness style i.e. an exercise

regimen without running, jumping and skipping. It is a combination of moves inspired by belly dance, Bollywood dance and African dance. It is actually a unique fitness technique that blends exercises from yoga, pilates, toning, body conditioning and mudra meditation etc.

History of Belly Fit

If we look back the history of bellyfit. It began in a small rural community in Ontario, Canada with the concept of renowned visionary dancer and entrepreneur Alice R. Bracegirdle in 2003. Initially, there were only fifteen naïve ladies in the groups to experience the bellyfit technique who had never danced before.

Later, groups of professionals, choreographers, mind and body specialists and musical visionaries have joined that group and promoted it across globe. Now, bellyfit is taught by hundreds of certified instructors across Canada- its origin place along with several other countries.

In India, it has emerged as a new fitness trend that is gaining popularity day by day. It is significantly liked and loved by ladies coming from different walks of life. Bellyfit instructors get intensive training to deliver a lesson in their class that offers an extraordinary full body exercise experience in a safe and effective way.

Yoga expert Jatinder Kumar says that bellyfit helps you to care about your entire being in an effective, safe and holistic manner.

Ashwini Ahuja

A Bellyfit for All Ages

Needless to say that bellyfit is for the ladies of all age groups, shapes and fitness levels. Generally, it is a six week health improvement programme for all. To join the class, you need not have any experience in dance and fitness practice is also not essential.

If you have the experience in belly dance, then bellyfit is more fun and ideal exercise for you. Bellyfit experts say that bellyfit class starts with a simple meditation followed by cardio session and then relax session.

This programme is split in two sessions. In the first session of half an hour, partakers burn calories, relieve their stress and let the sweat flowing and learn cardio moves by experiencing belly, Bollywood, Bhangra and African dance etc.

In the second session of bellyfit experience, they enjoy toning, sculpting and relaxing yoga in addition to mudra meditation. In a six week pleasant fitness programme, one aims to build stamina and improve strength having amazing stability and flexibility in the body. It also improves cardiovascular condition.

Yoga expert Jatinder Kumar says this programme has the similarity with the yoga. Like yoga, bellyfit also emphasizes the fluid movement of hips, abdomens, spine and shoulders, giving the buffs many benefits they simply won't get with simple running, jogging or exercise.

Jatinder Kumar further says that bellyfit is an intense cardio aerobics class with its core work. It is especially for mature female body. But if someone lady is pregnant, she should not join the bellyfit class because it would be dangerous for her as bellyfit requires hyper mobility in the joints, particularly in hips and pelvic region.

Health Benefits of Bellyfit

1. Bellyfit reduces body weight
2. It levels down the abdomen
3. It's a wonderful cardiovascular workout
4. It makes an improvement in posture
5. It makes the body flexible and supple
6. It detoxifies the body oozing sweat
7. Though bellyfit practice, ladies get rid of menstrual tension
8. It improves the digestive system
9. It builds a strong connection between the mind and the body
10. It helps in breath
11. It shapes the thighs and buttocks
12. It makes the back healthier
13. It makes the arms and shoulders leaner
14. It enables the ladies to cope with stress and pressure
15. It makes the mind calm and body relaxed
16. It gives a good feeling of feminine and sensuality
17. It releases stress and anxiety
18. It builds unbelievable confidence in ladies

Ashwini Ahuja

19   It tones their muscles around waistline

20   It's the only programme that brings together the mind, body and spirit.

Bellyfit Association with Chakras and Music

The health programme namely bellyfit is intensely associated with chakra and music. A chakra is a Sanskrit term meaning wheel. In a bellyfit class, the 'warm up' and the 'cool down' moves are related to chakras. These moves are especially designed to bring the participants' awareness to chakras and the muscles associated with them.

The simple formula is: when chakras are balanced, the body is balanced. When the body is balanced, the human being is also balanced and it shows the better result in health and beauty. And, the music is also very important feature in bellyfit class. It is the heart and the soul of the class experience. It is said that the sonic landscape which we hear in bellyfit class is nowhere found in any other group fitness class. The music- a fusion of an ethno fused techno, tribal rhythms and ambient tracks brings an energetic component to each class.

Nutritional Advice

If You Desire Best Result in Bellyfit Class

- ✓ Drink maximum water. Several times a day. It will flush out all of your toxins

- ✓ Avoid oily food. Prefer salads and green vegetables
- ✓ Avoid rice as much as you can
- ✓ Eat rotis that are not made in oil
- ✓ Drink green tea instead of black tea
- ✓ Avoid bakery items such as bread, bun etc
- ✓ Minimize the consumption of sugar and salt
- ✓ Eat food stuff rich in fiber beans, oat and almonds etc

A Fusion of Trio

In a nutshell, we can say that bellyfit is a blending of belly dance, yoga and fitness programme. It is a fusion of exercise, fun and art. Belly dance gives us graceful fluid moves, in the meanwhile massaging the internal organs. It shapes the waistline and increases body awareness. Moreover, belly dance lubricates the joints.

Yoga helps in joining together the mind, body and spirit. It improves the body posture, improves the body functions. Increase energy level. Improve health and flexibility. It strengthens the organs, build stamina and tones the body.

Chapter Two

For Perfect Body Shape

Healthy Diet and Regular Exercise

Ladies generally avoid wearing bikini when they head for a beach if they own extra flab on any part of their body. They are deprived of enjoying the happy sun and the sand of the sea.

If you are also one of such ladies and wearing swimming suit gives you nightmare only due to your extra flab or imperfect body shape, don't lose your heart and be depressed. Just remember only four precious words and tag on them forever.

The four words are: healthy diet, regular exercise. Believe, these four precious words will change the language and contour of your body and make you the 'beautiful darling' among friends. Experts say that inner thighs, love handles (*LOVE HANDLES* are the areas of skin that extend outward from the hips), back and triceps are most prominent places of the body for fat accumulation.

By doing regular exercise with balanced diets, you can get rid of it and give a good shape to your body making it charming and loving. Cardiovascular activities such as walking, jogging and stair climbing including a simple workout for every part of the body at least three days a week are necessary for good results but some precautions are necessary as well.

No Sweets, Only Fresh Fruits

If you have a good taste for sweets, don't binge on sweetmeats, pastries or ice creams etc. Opt for sweets in its natural form if you have a passion for sweet diets. Fresh fruits and berries are much better than sweetmeats. As for vegetables, they have a lot of vitamins and minerals. So, always prefer green, orange and yellow vegetables and necessarily avoid sugary and greasy snacks, chocolate, toffees and candies etc.

Nutritionist Geetu Amarnani says that green leafy vegetables are the best items to satiate your hunger. You can add some salads and soups with it to make better its taste. It will definitely help you in getting rid of extra inches on your waistline, getting you into an attractive shape. She further advises that health conscious ladies should avoid oily foods because that may make them feel bloated.

An Apple and a Lot of Water

Several nutritionists advise that an apple in the morning on regular basis is good to control the flab but remember- an apple means a full size apple, definitely not an apple pie. Moreover, drink water maximum in the morning regularly before setting out for an exercise. Bulgy thighs and sagging fat on the abs generally frighten the ladies. Fat on the abs is just like fat everywhere which gives the body an imperfect shape. So, water therapy is the best solution to reduce fat on abs.

Ashwini Ahuja

Dr. Anju Setia suggests that at least 10-12 glasses of water a day should be the necessity of the body to have desired results. Water in the early morning may detoxify you and help you in getting rid of accumulated salts.

Be alert that sugary soft drinks are not the substitute of water. If you are getting tired of plain water, you can add a slice of lemon or lime to give it a different taste but never substitute water with soft drinks or colas.

Food for Weight Loss

The present time is the age of fad foods. All fad foods are not unhealthy. There are several fad diets which will lead you to a successful weight loss provided you follow them exactly the same way as they are designed for.

After you learn which foods are good for you, you must get better your eating habits. The unhealthy eating habits are more dangerous than the food we eat. Have a look on healthy foods which may reduce weight and flab.

1   Leafy greens and lettuce
2   Fresh fruits and berries
3   Nut, dried fruits and healthy snacks
4   Canola and olive oils for cooking
5   Ocean fish
6   Seeds and legumes
7   Low fat milk and soya beverages

Undoubtedly, these foods are healthy but excess of calories is not good for you. So, be alert while consuming these foods also. You can also steam them to make its taste better and retaining the most nutritional value as well.

Avoid Saturated Fat

Our body needs a variety of foods to get all the vitamins and minerals we need for our healthy body. Generally, our diets are deficient in unsaturated fatty acids. So, it's much better if we take sea food two or three times a week.

Baked fish or chicken are healthier than fried. Processed diets such as hot dogs, bacon and red meats have a lot of fat and nitrates. So, avoid such foods.

Our body doesn't require such foods. If you have a love for these meats, you can take it in low quantity even its healthier version sold at branded food stores. Omega-3 foods such as flaxseed oil, avocados, olive oil, halibut, salmon, etc. are known best for reducing the flab. It must be included in your diet to give your body a shine and beauty.

Don't Destroy Skin Beauty

While exercising for body shape, don't forget that skin beauty is also important for attraction. Body shape and skin beauty always go together. So, be alert when you are out of the sea.

If you are not aware, salty water may harm your skin. Never let the saline water dry on your skin. Don't forget to take bath and moisture your skin once you are coming out of the sea. Don't forget to go for a deep conditioning treatment for hair after your come out of the sea.

And never ignore umbrella or cap for sun protection. Aloe Vera gel also helps in healing skin after sun exposure. Use it where and whenever you need it. Never destroy the glow of your skin. Without beauty skin, your body shape won't attract others.

Rajni Wadhwa, a beautician says that the ladies should use lotions not only on their face but all over their body. For extra protection, they can re-apply it after a gap of three four hours. They can protect their hair if they use any type of headgear or a cap before entering in the sea.

Treatment with Advance Technology

Moreover, in present time, technology is also here to help the ladies to get rid of the flab quickly. There are two types of technological treatments- non surgical and surgical. Non surgical treatment is called VIP complex. In this treatment, one has to spend almost Rs. 1000 to Rs. 3000 per session depending on the body structure and degree of the plump. Surgical treatment is called "Vibration Amplification of Sound Energy (VASER).

It is a costly treatment. One has to spend Rs. 50,000 to 150,000 depending upon the area to be covered. For this treatment, the planning for the one month is compulsory. Doctors say that it is better and quicker and less risk prone treatment for getting you into a finer shape.

In VASER treatment, the surgeon use ultrasonic sound waves to loosen up the flab accumulated in the body. VASER liposuction technology is beneficial in several ways in comparison to the traditional procedure. This advanced technique allows the surgeons to remove fat from the body with minimum risks and low impacts.

The best thing in this procedure is that it doesn't require general anesthesia. But, doctors suggest that ladies should think of the VASER technique if proper diet and exercise are no more effective on them.

Eat Smartly

Dieticians opine that healthy eating always begins with the concept of smart eating. It doesn't matter what you eat. It matters more how you eat. The health of anyone depends upon the choice of food and its ways of eating. Always remember that your food reduces the risk of heart diseases, cancer, TB, diabetes, blood pressure etc. If you know the habit of healthy eating, you can boost your energy; sharpen your memories and cheer up your mood.

Emotional eaters are always at more risk. Generally, most of the ladies engage in nibbling something while watching their favourite TV show. If you have the habit of crunching all the time, don't chew junk food like potato chips, ice cream and candies, all the time. You can munch green salad or fruits or oil free and moreover calorie free foods to satiate your hunger.

Ashwini Ahuja

No doubt, you may be a lover of chocolate or burger but be conscious, don't bring a pack of chocolates or pairs of burgers at home. Go to the market and enjoy eating what you wish. This way, you will devour less fast food.

Always remember that three time meals are essential to give energy to the body. Working women generally skip their breakfast due to busy schedule in the morning. Don't skip any meal. If you skip your breakfast, you may find that you are losing your energy by mid morning. Don't forget- a healthy breakfast can jumpstart your metabolism.

If you have no mood to take something in the morning, you may split it in half. You can eat an egg with a small diet of oatmeal to give required energy to your body. Some raisin and 10-15 pieces of almond are sufficient to eat in the midmorning.

Such diet is much better than taking some coffee with hot dog or burger at any eatery or coffee bar. Always take time to chew your food and savor every meal time. Always take small eating to keep your digestive system strong.

Exercise Zone

In exercise zone, you may include seven kinds of workout to give your body an attractive shape. These may be running, bicycling, cross country skiing, rowing, swimming, step aerobics, practice on elliptical trainer and kickboxing etc.

All these exercises are cardio activities. Needless to say that cardio is one of the most important things you need for your body. Whether it is the lose weight, improvement in the health or building the muscles, cardio is good for every body's part.

Running in the Ground

It is one of the best exercises for body shape and skin glow. In this exercise, you need not to spend anything on special equipment except some quality shoes. You can do this workout anytime and anywhere. Running will help you in building strong bones and connective tissues.

It will help you in burning serious calories also. It will get your heart rate up more quickly than any low or no impact exercise. By running about 30 minutes or less, you can burn at least three hundred calories.

By walk briskly the same time, you will find that you have burnt the half calories. By running continuously, you can also improve the strength of your stamina. Thus, running is quite good for having body shape.

Cross Country Skiing: An Incredible Workout

Gym expert Sanjeev Marshal opines that cross-country skiing is excellently an incredible cardio exercise. It doesn't matter either you are on a gym machine or swooshing over snow.

In cross country skiing, both the upper and the lower parts of the body have to work. Skiing just half an hour burns about 350 calories. It is a wonderful workout for body shape and its wellbeing.

Use the Power of Legs

Ashwini Ahuja

Cycling is also an excellent cardio workout. It helps a lot to shape the body. It is not necessary to go out of home for cycling. In your home gym, you can use the power of your legs on stationary bicycle. Cycling increases endurance while burning a lot of calories.

Within thirty minutes of cycling, one can burn 250-300 calories depending on you how fast you run cycle and how high your resistance is.

The best point in cycling is that you can use it while going to your workplace also. Cycling is a low impact exercise. It is good for joints also. Cycling is just like running or aerobics.

Exercise on Elliptical Trainer

Like treadmill, elliptical trainer is also a machine which is most popular for cardio workout. Every gym owns an elliptical trainer. This machine allows the body to move in a natural way without the impact of treadmill. One can add intensity by increasing resistance.

This machine is a good choice for runners looking for a break from pounding the ground. One can do muscle exercise in a different way on elliptical trainer. By doing exercise on elliptical trainer, a person can burn 300 calories within thirty minutes.

Fun in the Water

Swimming is not only an exercise but a fun for you also. Like cross country skiing, it's another great choice for cardio exercise. In fact, swimming is a full body exercise. The more parts you involve in the exercise, the more calories you will burn and give more good shape to your body.

By doing breaststrokes for just thirty minutes, you can burn more than 400 calories. In swimming, you have no risk of injuries as joints are fully supported to the body. In fact, swimming is the best exercise for body shape.

Step Aerobics

Step aerobics is also a calories burner workout. It targets our legs, hips and butt etc. By doing step aerobics, one can burn at least 300- 400 calories. Moreover, aerobics is very easy to learn. It's not just a workout but a fun also.

For those people who like choreographed workouts, step aerobics is one of the best exercises for them. One can learn step aerobics at home with the help of video.

Exercise with Rowing Machine

Exercise on rowing machine is often overlooked in the gym. Generally, sports persons visiting the gym are confused over the working of rowing machine. They don't know how a rowing machine delivers a great workout.

In fact, rowing, at present, is a physically demanding exercise that involves both the upper and lower part of the body. Exercise on rowing machine burn more calories than several other exercises.

Ashwini Ahuja

Like a stationary bicycle or an elliptical trainer, there are different levels of resistance which allows you to get a challenging workout no matter what your fitness level.

Half an hour exercise on rowing machine burns at least 300 calories. At start, rowing is a tough exercise. If you are new and never tried rowing, you may feel difficulty.

In this situation, you can start your day with 10-15 minutes on rowing machine. Later, you can add more time to subsequent workouts according to the requirement of your body. The final word is: none can deny the importance of rowing exercise in shaping your body.

You won't be able to shape your body if you....

- ✓ Eat greasy snacks or something like that in front of TV without giving it much thought
- ✓ Start eating when you are sad, bored or happy
- ✓ Prefer your meals at restaurants in stead of taking meals at home
- ✓ Love to relish fast food regularly
- ✓ Skip breakfast or lunch carelessly and then overeat at night
- ✓ Crave for sweetmeats, pastries, ice creams, soft drinks, white bread, refined pasta and oily snacks etc.

Chapter Three

Make Living Room Stylish

Do you know living room in the house reflects aesthetic quotient? It is one of the busiest and multi-utility rooms in the house accommodating the dining set, the TV, fridge etc.

All the members of the family collect in this room from time to time to have fun, play indoor games, watch TV; dine together and meeting guests.

It is the place in the house which actually mirrors the lifestyle so it definitely should be kept neat and clean so as it may serve as a comfortable and fine place for everyone to sit and relax.

Delhi based interior designer Payal Gupta says that one can transform living room into a luxury and dream room with the blending of imagination, creativity and elegant taste. She further says that in recent times, due to hike in real estate prices, spaces have become constricted so it is need of the time; we utilize the space to the full.

Now-a-days, in many homes, people prefer to build an open kitchen on the side in the living room without disturbing its visual appeal. With the right balance of colours and textures, we can make our living room excellent which exhibits class and elegance. Here are some ideas which may be helpful for decorating the living room.

- Arrange the furniture of your living room in such a way that it doesn't block the traffic of the room. It will give the living room a neat look. Make sure to have sufficient space for moving inside the room also.

Don't place decorative items in the walk way. The way from main door to living room should be unhindered by any of the domestic item.

Don't block windows with books and domestic items. Make sure the room has plenty of sunlight and cool breeze which not only will brighten the room but make its appearance larger.

The use of mirrors in the living room also visually gives the look larger. They make the room pleasing and elegant so; use the mirrors on either side of the room.

Green plants add fragrance and colour to the living room. They give the room a natural and cool look. Artificial plants also can be kept for decoration. Arrange them in colourful vases.

By painting one wall of the room and leaving the other walls unpainted, you can give the living room a sophisticated look.

You can choose either bold or contrasting colours or lighter or subtle ones, it entirely depends on your choice.

Any change in colours will definitely give your living room an arresting look.

Attractive and chic lamps can also be placed in the room to heighten its look.

You can place them either on the side table or the floor.

If you have antique pieces- such as grandfather clock, mirror cabinet, timbered chair coming from your grandparents, show off them in your living room.

Trophies, mementoes also can be showcased on mantelpiece. It will give your personality a grace without spending even a penny.

Photo frames having your family photographs, kids' photos and work of art can also be displayed at the mantelpiece.

Decoration of greeting cards can also be hung in any corner of the living room.

Books too are decorative pieces. Coffee table books add great value to the centre table of the living room.

Last but not least, never try to overdo. Your living room should look like a comfort zone, not an art gallery or any hotel.

Avoid overcrowding. Never make your living room cluttered and disorganized.

Chapter Four

Be Attractive In the Party

You must have observed that in some wedding parties or other get-together celebrations, generally those ladies are getting more noticed who look quite different from the crowd because of their gorgeous dress, beauteous and ravishing smile, scintillating jewelry, attractive hairstyles and the impressive manner of their conversation with friends or relatives etc.

It is not necessary you should have been ravishing beautiful to attract others. If you are sober and simply fine-looking lady, you can also register your presence in the party with your exclusive style. Learn some tips how you can get noticed by several guys.

Improve Your Posture

Most ladies don't understand the importance of posture. It is the first and one of the most important points to enhance the personality. Remember, bad posture will make the look depressed, uninterested and purely homely woman. None may want to stand near you only due to your unimpressive posture. So, when you are attending a party, you must be aware of your right posture.

Don't slouch excessively. Discard your fear and hesitation. If you have the habit of making such posture at home, do it correct forthwith by health exercises for the back. You get down on the floor and think of your back as a table. Put your knees under your hips and hands under your shoulders. Pull your tummy in but keep the back straight. Such types of exercise at home definitely will improve your posture.

So, don't forget to correct it as early as possible. Never pose it in the party. Moreover, place your head straight on the top of your neck. Make sure; your shoulders are upright and back is arched forward.

In such posture, you will look taller and even greatly confident. Leave your arms relaxed and unstressed. Remember, the right posture will keep you active and energetic throughout the day also.

Ravishing & Beauteous Smile

It is true that the ladies who walk around flashing a ravishing and beauteous smile are always perceived to be more attractive and charming, so; always make your smile brightly fulsome and win the hearts of people you meet in the party.

It is also quite true that a healthy smile reflects the mood and the personality and displays our inner health and beauty. Smiling faces make the others happier and give them warm invitation for having constant relationship. It makes the bond stronger with others. Moreover, smiling and laughing make you look younger and it will boost your spirits too.

It is not surprising that some ladies may ask how they can improve their smile. It is quite simple. You can improve your smile by doing practice in front of the mirror. Remember, nice teeth are the cornerstone of a ravishing smile. Be sure your teeth are shinning white. If they are not, pay your attention towards them and make them whitened to make your smile brightening.

Visit the dentist if it is necessary for it or get prescription telephonically. Also, don't let become your smile as a smirk. It may disrepute you.

Get Groomed Yourself

To make your presence prominent in any party, get yourself fully groomed. First of all, get rid of all unwanted hair on your body. Unwanted hair gives a bad look to the body. They include ear, nose, face, arms and legs hair etc. Don't forget to pluck an unwanted hair on your eyebrows also.

Most ladies visit beauty parlors for threading on eyebrows before they attend to any function. Only eliminating an eyebrow makes a change in the looks of their face. Imagine how you look great when all of your arms and legs are sleek, soft and hairless. Apart from it, don't forget to do other actions such as trimming of the nails and cleaning the wax out of your ears.

Do control your acne, dandruff and other skin's bad conditions if it happens. Get yourself fully groomed and be the queen of the party.

Let the Dance Show Your Charisma

In wedding party, the girls and the ladies who dance generally attract the all attentions; even they attract the attention of the opposite sex more. In marriage parties, dance groups of danseuse girls are hired to entertain the guests.

Undoubtedly, they are perceived to be more sexual and people notice them casually despite a few drunkards hover around them but if a guest lady dance individually, she is noticed more and is respected as a special guest.

Hosts too pay more respect and attentions to such guests and treat them specials. So, if you are naturally a good dancer, it is okay. If you are not, attend a few dance classes and learn the skill so as to show your presence in the party with your dancing skill and earn respect. Let the individual-dance show your charisma in the party.

Believe, individual dance is always wonderful; you will see what kind of response you get when you are getting bopped onto the dancing floor individually in the party.

Exclusive Hair-Cut

To get yourself noticed especially, your haircut also needs to be exclusively great and good-looking, and for it; before you attend the wedding party; you must visit any renowned saloon where the bigwigs and the movie stars prefer to visit.

No doubt, such saloons are expensive but it is the one time deal and definitely it is not more costly than your charisma which you are intending to show in the party. Think- why movies stars look different. They look different because they spend money lavishly to look different and make what they like, with their appearance.

Stylists know how to shape a haircut around your face. First, they observe the type of the face and the size of the head etc. then make the hair-cut attractive and quite different to all others.

Pea-cocking With Accessories

Have you ever heard about the "Pea-cocking" term? It is best known for all those fashion stylists who purposefully dress themselves in such a fascinating way so as they could draw others' attention in the gatherings.

Most celebrities wear different types of accessories such as long earrings, hats, necklaces, glasses, scarves, watches, bracelets and belts etc. along with their fine outfits to attract others' attentions.

Accessories are such items which increase the sparkle of wearer's outfit more. With the good use of such accessories you can also make yourself noticeable in the crowd. To make the appearance glitzy, in the party; peacock yourself with the varieties of accessories.

Smell Good to Magnetize Others

Using perfume is also a good way to attract others in the party particularly the men. Men are generally more attracted to scented women because the fragrance releasing from women's body encourage them to stay longer in their company and it makes their emotions intensely strong.

Needless to say that smell in itself is one of the brain's strongest senses so, the better you smell the more attractive you will be appearing to others; not only to men but the other ladies also.

The investment in buying a good cologne or perfume is a wise step to crowd people around you. Remember one important point, when you buy a brand perfume, you must seek men's opinion in your friends' circle to ensure its results.

Also, make sure, you always put the right amount of the scent on you. Too much of its use can turn the others off from you.

Chapter Five

Perk up Mood

Life is not a bed of only roses. It is a mixture of both roses and thorns. Sometimes, in our life, we, due to some unwanted reasons, feel depressed, low and sad. We then try our best to find a way to get relaxed but desperately remain failed. In reality, none in life wants to be tensed and disturbed. Here are some ways that will help you cheer up your mood.

Think positively

Things are the same but it is the perception that matters. If you think positive and also do positive, you will get positive response in return from others. Look at the glass which is half full as well as half empty. It depends on you how you take it, positive or negative?

If you take it negative, you will burn up yourself, if you take it positive; happiness and hope will smile on you. Read self-help books which are generally for "point up" how to sway your mood swings.

The attitude of optimism is essential for the elevation of mood which comes with the reading the books on optimism.

Don't Suppress Feelings

Why are you unhappy and melancholic? Try to find out the actual reasons. Don't suppress your feelings. Share your thoughts with friends, colleagues, family members and near and dear. Try to be happy forever and enjoy the every moment. Be resolute. Don't allow gloom enter in your life ever.

Reconnect with Nature

The beauty of nature makes the sad persons happy and delighted. It helps in mood enhancement. So, always try to reconnect with green nature. Go for a regular stroll and enjoy nature's greenery. Listening to the chirps of birds will also make you refresh pepping up your mood.

Avoid Unnecessary Stress and Tension

Avoid stress as much as possible. Be relaxed, carefree and unworried. Take life as it comes naturally avoiding unnecessary tension for the reasons of both your personal and professional life.

Sound Sleep

Sound mind lives in a sound body. Body becomes sound when we sleep soundly. So, never sacrifice your sound sleep. Sleep at least 6 hours daily is essential to get you relaxed, fit and healthy.

If you feel relaxed, your mood will automatically be happy. You must have heard people become cranky due to lack in sound sleep. Insomnia or disturbed sleep makes us distraught and depressed.

Healthy Breakfast

Have you ever thought about the food you eat? It also decides your mood. So, start your day with healthy and nutritious breakfast. You may be busy or late for the office. Maybe you miss the train which ferries you to workplace but never skip breakfast whatever the reasons maybe. It will not affect your health but mood also. Take your favourite carb in breakfast that will make your mood lively.

According to some researches, chocolates also can help you relax and enhance your mood. Try on it if its taste delights you. Last but not least, simple mantra to perk up your mood is: remember the above tips and follow it smilingly.

Chapter Six

Passion for Silver Jewellery

Every woman loves to wear precious gold. Also, she dreams of wearing dazzling diamond but in recent times, she has an ardent passion for silver jewellery as well.

In view of its cost and variety, silver jewellery attracts the ladies of all ages even more as they can experiment with their choice and style without worrying about the puncture in your pockets. Silver jewellery is available in all types from the ankle or waist to the rings, bangles, bracelets, chains, armlets; toe rings, nose rings apart from the necklace and the earrings etc.

It is known for its aesthetic value. It is rather more popular among funky college girls. Women can wear it with sari, skirt, salwar-kameez or even jeans etc. In recent times, designers are keen on designing simple, sober, lightweight and unique silver jewellery to charm women customers. Silver jewellery, at present, is quite different from the old time bulky silver jewellery and is available in the market with different temperaments and styles.

Both working women and housewives love to wear it as their pet accessories. If you want to beautify your personality economically and elegantly then silver jewellery may be your best option.

Indeed, the versatility in silver jewellery attracts the women. Wearing silver jewellery is considered a modern simple fashion among fashionable girls and sophisticated ladies. They prefer light and comfy jewellery so as not to get exhausted during their hectic daily routines but women living in both rural and tribal areas prefer to heavy silver jewellery to adorn themselves.

It also gives them financial security during contingency apart from determining their marital status as well as the community the women belong to, by their wearing style.

Youngsters in cities can also be noticed adorning themselves with silver jewelry as a fashion. Connoisseurs say that the trend of making new silver jewellery by melting the old ones is prevalent across the globe apart from India.

In India, silver jewellery is made at Kolhapur (Maharashtra); Salem (Tamil Nadu), Hathras (UP) and Rajkot (Gujarat) etc. but it is worn tastefully by women living in all parts of the country.

Traditionally, in old times, the women of Gujarat, Rajasthan, Andhra Pradesh and north-eastern states loved to wear it profusely. It was then adorned by both men and ladies. Ladies wore it to boost up their beauty and men adorned it as a symbol of power and strength. Even today, men too love wearing it stylishly.

Some women generally complain that silver jewellery is not better than the gold coated artificial jewellery because it gets oxidized within short period and loses its gleam.

No doubt, Indian climate is an arch enemy of silver if you are absolutely careless. Designers advisably emphasis that silver jewellery must be cleaned time to time maintaining its sparkle as generally it is combined with copper (approximately 7.5 percent) which makes it hard and retains its shape so it is very essential you apply proper cleaning solution to your jewellery.

First of all, always store the jewellery in the jewellery box. It is tarnished due to reaction between the oxygen, silver and sulphur so put it off while you go for swimming, bathing or washing.

Be careful also while you applying for hair spray. If tarnish develops due to some inadvertent reasons, use the simple procedure of boiling jewellery in a solution of sodium chloride and sodium bicarbonate.

Ashwini Ahuja

Chapter Seven

Make the Day Special

Wedding day is the special time in the life of every girl and she wants to be at her best appearance on that day. She dreams to look like a fabulous princess of the event but all girls are not so lucky to make this day marvelous

The wedding season comes every now and then in India. It is the time for every bride-to-be to get ready herself on this very special and big day. Every girl wants to look most beautiful on this day. No doubt, professional make-up artist and beauticians try their best to make the bride superlative, the dream girl of bridegroom but it is equally important to remember that the health and skin care and also the diet of the bride is as important as make-up preparations or marriage arrangements to crown her the queen of the event.

Several days before the ceremony which is known as a mega event of the family, the bride-to-be has to make several tasks and shopping assignments, so, the sleepless nights and disturbed eating before the wedding makes her so tired that her skin looks dull and face stressed. Lack of energy and the trouble of indigestion are commonplace problems every wedding girl has to cope with.

Certainly, wedding day is of greater importance in the life of any girl. All girls enthusiastically wait for this special day. Here are some tips for bride-to-be to make her day great, memorable and wonderful.

Skin Care is Essential

At least a month before the special day, the bride should start caring about her skin so that she may look more pretty, attractive, gorgeous, fresh and most beautiful on the day of her marriage. Health experts opine that fresh juice, green vegetables and fruits and a lot of water get the skin to look young, exquisite, attractive and bright. Always keep yourself tension free. Morning walk is also one of the best tools to have the glow of the skin. Massage of oil or body lotion also makes the skin relaxed and lustrous.

Rajni Wadhwa, a beautician says that minimum 15 days before the marriage, every girl should apply the packs of lemon, haldi, (turmeric) sandalwood and beson (gram flour) with the mix of rose water or milk on her body to pep up the skin.

Before applying mixture, cleansing of the skin is very essential. After some time, the girl should wash her face with cold water to avoid wrinkles. Attractive nails increase the beauty of fingers. So, it is very essential to rub olive oil on nails in round movement.

Rajni Wadhwa further suggests that on the day of marriage, the eyes of the bride-to-be should also look fresh and clear. For this purpose, they should put 2-3 drops of rose water into their days two times a day.

It is the best method to make the eyes fresh and charming. Rajni concludes that good eating habits and

Ashwini Ahuja

regular exercise are as important to the skin health as they are totally body health.

Make Your Hair Shiny and Silky

It is well said that beautiful hair is brides' crowning glory. Before the day of wedding, make sure, your hairs look shiny and silky. Overall, you are the queen of your special day. Be alert; don't let tresses make fun of you. The mixture of amla, shikakai, egg, reetha (soap nut) and tea water makes the hairs lustrous, silky and smooth.

Apply this mixture regularly almost half a month before the wedding day. Leave the mixture just a day before the wedding. You will wow to see the amazing results. The hair style always matters. Remember that the perfect hair style will make your look more charming and elegant. For it, you need to make prior appointments with your beautician so that she may do a proper hair care regime.

Generally, brides allow their beautician or stylist to pull the hairs back tightly to set right them for long hours. Hairs are your precious assets; don't let anyone play with them. The exercise will end up with a severe headache and ruin the cherished moments of your wedding's delight and charm. If it is necessary, you may practice hairstyle with your hands instead.

Hair stylists take care of brides' hair after identifying its nature. There are generally three types of hair- normal, oily and dry. The care of the hair depends upon the type of hair. Natural care of the hair is always good. It has proved that the excessive use of blow dryers and synthetic colours spoil the texture of hair and damage it forever. Harsh chemicals deprive its natural sheen.

Sun light is also harmful for the shine of hair. Over exposure to sun light may discolour the hair tips. At least a month before the wedding day, if you have to step out for some essential work, make sure that your hair should be covered with some cloth or a cap. Combing the wet hair also spoil its shine. Always let your hair dry before combing and brushing it. Always use wide tooth wooden brush for combing.

Lips and Nails Care

Lips and nails of the bride are also an attraction for others. The more you outlined the lips, the more they will attract other and make your smile beauteous. So, to make your lips charming, you need to take a few extra steps. Before applying lip colour, smooth a bit of foundation over your lips. It will make your lipstick more evenly and allow it stay longer.

Ask your beautician to outline the lips with a lip liner then fill in lips with the liner. With the help of lip brush, also apply one coat of lip colour. Use tissue paper to remove the blot if it appears around the lips. Then, apply the second coat of lip colour. Come what may, make lips charming and always smiling. Let the colour of lips glow with your wedding smile.

As for the nails, every bride wants to look them perfect on dream day. Her henna decorated hands and polished nails also attract the visitors. The first thing about the nails is that they must be mar-free. If you have the habit of biting nails, now it is the time for you to stop this unpleasant practice. Generally, guests and ladies want to observe the wedding/engagement rings of the bride. The decorated hands of the brides are also videographed.

So, the nails of the bride necessarily should look best. You can use a nail strengthener to ensure hands look beautiful for special day. Rajni Wadhwa, beautician says that fingernails take thirty minutes to dry completely so, be more careful first half an hour after applying the polish on your nails.

Some girls are allergic to nail polish. If you have also any type of allergy with the nail polish, you should tell the beautician to have a manicure without polish. By having manicure, your cuticles will look nice and neat. Tell the beautician to buff your nails.

Don't forget, a day before the wedding, you must have a professional manicure. On the day of wedding; you may be asked to have numerous close-up photos of your hands.

Rajni Wadhwa says that French manicure is good for such occasions. It gives a natural look. Always remember that if you are planning to have black and white photographs, you need to change your makeup. Soft colours generally don't show up well in black and white photographs. For black and white pictures, you should wear more intense and neutrals and darker lipsticks.

Care about Diet

Always remember that pre-wedding health is not all about weight loss and pseudo spa treatments. It is the time for the brides to be to stay healthy and make her shape attractive before walking down the *mandap.* (pavilion)

Dr. Amit Sachdeva says that taking a healthy diet before the marriage is important, not only for the bride, but it is equally important for the groom also. The diet of the bride should be more nutritious than groom as per the need of her body. Vitamin C, Vitamin A, Vitamin E and proteins are essential for bride.

Balanced diet will cheer up her mood and make the auspicious occasion delightful. Before the two three months of the wedding, the girls should be conscious about their health. The three main meals of the day are necessary for the wellbeing of health of the girl despite that she has been planning to reduce her weight.

Dr. Amit Sachdeva further says that a marriageable girl needs at least 1600 calories. In health science, for such girls, three times meals are recommended. If you are going to be married shortly, never skip the breakfast. It is necessary to start a day with healthy diet. You must include fibre, proteins, and carbohydrates in breakfast. Fresh fruits, juice, milk oatmeal, soya, cheese etc. are compulsory for would-be-brides.

Ashwini Ahuja

Soft drinks, soda, alcohol, excess of coffee and tea should be avoided. Like breakfast, the lunch should also be completely nutritious for the bride i.e. high in fibre, vitamins, minerals and proteins etc. Dr. Amit Sachdeva suggests that well balanced lunch is good for health that keeps the bride active for the most part of the day. For marriageable girls, the third meal of the day – dinner should be light and low in calories because the body needs low calories at the time of sleep. Bride should avoid fried foods, polished rice, breads and high calories drinks at the time of sleep.

For the good health and wellbeing of the body, drinking water at least 10-15 glasses is necessary. It will hydrate the body and give an amazing shine to your skin. Apart from balanced diet, regular exercise is also very important. For boosting hair growth, you need to take in Omega 3 enriched food like fishes and green vegetables and sprouts etc. It is equally important for the bride to stay away from all types of stresses to enjoy the special day.

Beauty Line: A Day before the Nuptial Day

1. Make an appointment with the beautician a day before marriage.
2. Make the appointment in the morning hours to have facial, manicure, pedicure or body massage so as you may get a time for relax.
3. Take a long bath a day before and the also day of event
4. Always remain stress free
5. Eat small meals. Heavy meals may affect your health

6   Take deep breaths if any sort of worry assails on you. Deep breaths will drive out the worries.

7   Practice dressing up at least a day before the ceremony. Ask your beautician to be available on your guard for necessary make-up touches. Practice the make up before hand is quite necessary

8   Don't colour your hair the day of wedding. Do such tasks in advance at least one day before the wedding

9   Keep blotting papers with you for its use time to time. It is necessary to absorb the perspiration

10   Shop your honeymoon clothes and trousseau before the day of event

11   Don't stay up late to plan the wedding. Lack of sleeplessness may ruin your health.

Essential Regular Work Out

For the wellbeing of mind and good health; exercise and yoga are necessary for the bride. Different types of workouts make the body fit and mind strong. You may accompany a friend while going for gym or ground. Doing exercise alone is a bored activity. It would be much better if you exercise with your friend.

The company of a friend will keep you motivated and on the right track. Remember that your exercise routine should be fun, not a chore. You should add music with your workout routine. Some ladies prefer brisk walk as an essential workout.

No doubt, walking is a good exercise. It not only helps you make your mind strong and relieve stress but also burn more calories. If you too have such planning, first of all, you need to find a right pair of shoes for it. It depends on you whether you choose high impact casual shoes or low impact sports shoes but remember that your shoes should be able to absorb the shock and keep your joints free from stress.

As for the exercise, wear clothes what you feel comfortable. They should let you breathe properly. Some ladies have 'curved posture' that curtail the elegance and beauty of the bride, so; always learn the habit of standing up straight. Good posture makes you look more attractive. For good posture, you can practice yoga in the supervision of yoga expert also.

Workout outfits should not be like fashion clothing. They must signify the fitness statement. Do exercise regularly but don't let it become obsessive. Exercise is meant for enhance the life, don't rule it your life.

The last but most important point: if you have the fear your menstrual cycle coincides with your wedding day, don't be careless in making an appointment with the doctor to sort out this biggest problem.

Last words

Always remember that a happy bride is a healthy bride. Healthy woman attracts her groom and make her wedding moments memorable and extremely enjoyable. So, always be positive and enjoy the ride of your newly wed life.

Don't be casual about anything for your preparation making the event meaningful and excellent. Remember that the day of wedding comes once in life. It is always a special day so, enjoy your day with fullness of happiness.

Chapter Eight

Organic Clothes for Family

These days, people are more conscious about their lifestyle. So, the demand for eco-friendly organic garments is higher than before. Apparently, it is due to our fear for global warming in the eco system. To meet the soaring demand, organic stuff has hit the fashion industry. Needless to say that organic clothing is not just limited to the youngsters only, it is liked by all - kids, women and professionals also as these clothes allow the skin to breathe better. For babies, they are more advantageous as they allow the moisture to evaporate making the skin of the baby softer and fresher the whole day,

No doubt, organic fabrics and clothing are better than other normal garments' stuff. They are made from materials such as cotton, wool, jute, silk and bamboo. Organic clothes are totally free from harmful chemicals which make the skin allergic to some types of toxic substances if we wear non-organic clothes.

Health expert Sanjeev Marshal says that wearing organic clothes means always making your skin allergy free and keeps the doctors away. Moreover, organic fibers are more durable and superior in quality. They last for more than one hundred machine washes before the fibers begin to chunk.

Organic clothes are more helpful for the environment in several ways also.

What is Organic Clothing?

Organic clothing is made from natural production of cotton, bamboo, silk, wool, jute etc. which is grown without using artificial or synthetic substances. The farming and processing that work with nature and help minimize air, soil and water pollution is known as organic farming and clothes made from such produces are known organic clothes.

Generally, artificial or toxic pesticides are used to protect the cotton or bamboo crops. The clothes made from such crops are not organic. If you are health conscious, never buy such unauthentic, so-called organic clothes.

Any labelled organic product, whether it's a tee shirt or ladies' outfit has to meet the national standards set by the United States Department of Agriculture. First of all, check their standards. If they seem genuine, then buy.

Organic Clothes are Environment Friendly

It has scientifically proved that organic clothing contributes to the well being of our environment. Organic clothes have anti-bacterial properties. They don't hold on to odour. Organic clothes made from bamboo or cotton fibers are two degrees lower than normal garments in hot weathers as well as warm in cold seasons. Such clothes give the body a soft and supple touch. Not only in India, the organic clothes are liked and dressed in Britain, Japan, USA, Canada, China and several other countries also.

Ashwini Ahuja

Due to health benefits, its' popularity is increasing day by day. One of the bad effects of organic cloth is that it develops wrinkles just by a single wearing or hanging in the closet. So, you need permanent ironing before wearing them. After ironing, however, a good quality cotton shirt looks much better than any other garment that you washed and hung.

Designers say that these days, non-organic cotton is developed by using several kinds of fertilizers and pesticides. Very often, a special kind of chemical substance formaldehyde is also used to give quality to cloth stuff. No doubt, formaldehyde stops wrinkles in cotton clothes, but this substance is a cancer causing agent and it is very harmful to wear such cotton clothes.

Best for New Born Infant

Organic clothes are the best and the safest to use for new born babies. The new born babies are delicate, soft and sensitive like flowers, so organic clothes don't annoy their skin like the non organic clothes.

Moreover, the babies don't have the developed immunity to harmful chemicals like adults, so, the synthetic fibres or additives are dangerously more harmful to the soft skin of the babies. With organic clothes, the babies won't ingest harmful chemicals whenever they playfully nibble the collars of their shirts.

Dr. Amit Sachdeva says that the skin of the baby is thinner and less oily than the skin of an adult. So, it is easy for that skin to absorb things quickly. Moreover, the skin of the baby produces less melanin which is a good substance to help the child from sunburn.

Dr. Anju Setia of Rajasthan says that babies sweat less than the adults. So, it's more difficult for them to maintain the inner temperature of the body. Needless to say, that choosing organic clothes for children cut down their exposure to toxins.

Why We Should Prefer Organic Clothes

Organic clothes are good for health. They are made of the stuff which is produced naturally without the use of chemicals or pesticides. Organic fabric is softer than non-organic products. It is an antibacterial and hypoallergenic product. It absorbs the moisture quickly and keeps the body dry and adour-free. Organic clothes made from bamboos can dry quickly.

It is surprising to hear but it is true that clothes made from bamboo release a significant amount of oxygen into the atmosphere. Bamboo fabric is created from bamboo pulp. It is bleached without the use of chlorine. So, it is much better if we prefer organic clothes.

Organic Clothes are Yoga Friendly

Needless to say, that; organic clothes are comfortable and totally chemical free clothes, so they are best outfits for yoga session. Yoga expert Jatinder Kumar says that by wearing organic clothes, not only you will be protecting the environment but you may speedily improve your health also. Organic clothes are sweat-absorbent. By wearing such clothes means that you always will be free of the sticky feeling while you are in an exercise or in a yoga mode. It has also proved that chemically processed fabrics generally cling to the body but the organic clothes don't stick. They keep the sweat off the body.

Yoga expert Jatinder Kumar further says that organic clothes are not only health friendly, they are nature-friendly also. They keep the smell off your nose. Undoubtedly, organic clothes are made from grown plants carefully without the use of chemical. So, they are costlier than common non organic or synthetic clothes but always keep in mind that you will get more the money by getting health benefits and the quality for what you pay in buying such clothes.

All Cotton is Not Organic

Some people think that cotton is naturally an organic production but it is not true. There is a lot of difference between the natural cotton and the organic cotton.

Despite the fact that cotton is natural and natural things are eco-friendly but it is subjected to different processes before it is ready to be used. When cotton is converted into cotton clothes, cotton is heavily processed. Several types of chemicals and toxins are used.

As a result, it is stripped of the natural waxes found in the material. On the other hand, organic cotton clothing is produced without the use of pesticides and fertilizers. For organic products, natural colours and dyes are used. These clothes are totally free from harmful toxins and colours.

Thus, we should understand the difference between the cotton and organic cotton. Non organic clothing is not eco friendly. When wearing such clothes, the toxic chemicals absorb into our skin and harm our respiratory system. Moreover, the residues of conventionally grown cotton may cause asthma, fatal poisoning and cancer also.

Why the Organic Clothes are Necessary

- ✓ They are toxin free.

- ✓ They are free from most dangerous chemical formaldehyde.

- ✓ They are very easy on the human skin.

- ✓ We feel incredibly comfortable by wearing them.

- ✓ They are known best for health and our respiratory system.

- ✓ They are sturdier than non organic.

- ✓ No pesticides and harmful substances are used.

- ✓ They are good for both our kids and family and the environment.

- ✓ They support true economy.

- ✓ If we wear them, we may help in protecting farm workers and quality of the water in addition to soil erosion.

- ✓ They are hypoallergenic.

Ashwini Ahuja

✓ They are useful for people with sensitive skin.

✓ They don't cause skin allergies or reactions.

✓ They destroy bacteria.

✓ In organic clothes, natural colours are used which don't fade easily.

✓ Organic clothes have natural sheen and oil of natural fabric.

✓ Organic clothes block UV rays and wicks moisture from the skin.

Hard Facts about Non Organic Clothing

1   In producing just one pair of jeans and T shirt, one pound of pesticides and chemical fertilizers are used.

2   During the conversion process of conventional cotton into clothing several toxic chemicals such as ammonia, formaldehyde, flame and soil retardants and petroleum scours etc. are used.

3   Formaldehyde is a harmful chemical (cancer agents) that is used in the manufacture of non organic clothes also

Finally

In a nutshell, we can say that organic clothes are better for our family and kids because organic cotton is grown by using methods and materials that have a low impact on our environment. By growing organic produce, we help to maintain soil fertility also.

And moreover, we help in building a more biologically diverse agricultural system. The best and easiest way to support organic clothing is our shopping. Think first, if you love your kids and family, if your answer is in a positive mode, start avoiding buy the non organic clothes.

Happily, go for organic clothes which are far away from chemicals and harmful artificial agents.

Ashwini Ahuja

Chapter Nine

Party Decorum

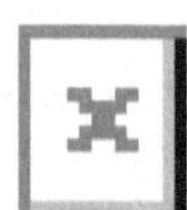

Parties or festivities are obviously an occasion to celebrate the moments of happiness for both the guests and the host. In wedding or engagement parties, we, in general, meet with friends, relatives and family members. Decorum, host's individual care for every guest and etiquettes make the celebration a decent and fabulous congregation.

Socialist Alok Srivastva opines that if you are organizing an engagement or wedding party, you should be more alert because it is the different from other social gatherings as it ties two different families in a connubial bond. Engaged or married couples and their parents and siblings keep the memories of such parties alive in their entire life. Celebration or party is an intimate affair which involves close friends and families.

Choose Sophisticated Venue

Although, there is no hard and fast rule regarding the venue of the celebration yet customarily, most families prefer to organize engagement parties or marriage parties at their farmhouse, club, resort or marriage palaces. Both the families- the family of bride and the groom- these days- jointly host the party.

No matter, where it takes place, but, to maintain the decorum, always choose calm, serene and fully decorated area facilitating the guests of different moods.

Mrs. Mamta Jain, a newly wed woman says that now-a-days, couples themselves take the responsibility to organize the party and it is a good of them in sharing the interests and developing the sense of understanding between them.

Decoration Gives Elegance

Mrs. Mamta Jain emphasizes, it is the host or hostess who is completely accountable if the party meets failure and all the credit also goes to them if it becomes a success. Its mode entirely depends on your fancy or needs. You can either organize luncheon or dinner party but if you love to enjoy the moments, prefer the night parties.

Night party gives more elegance to the ceremony. If you are organizing night party, don't forget to decorate the venue with strings of fairy lights and electric candles etc. to create a romantic atmosphere.

Mrs. Mamta further says that it might be utterly ugly if we let go the moments of romance waste in an unromantic atmosphere.

Ashwini Ahuja

Guests' Listing

The guests are the grace of every party. The host/hostess feels proud meeting nice, sober and elegant guests at the party venue but always be heedful about guests' list. If the groom family visits bride's home with some 50 guests, the family of the bride should not invite guests in hundreds. It will look awkward.

So, plan the short as well as the long list carefully and separately also. Those guests whom you are going to invite in the upcoming marriage, you must invite them in engagement party also.

Horde of garrulous friends and relatives sometimes make the party a place of hullabaloo. Be observant and eliminate the cacophony of the noises with your best possible efforts. Send the invitations to guests at least a week earlier as some people are sluggish and take awhile to react.

It is better if we visit guests' home personally to invite them. If it is not possible, don't forget to ring them and remind of the party after sending the invitation cards to them.

Respect the Guests Individually

As being a host or hostess, make sure that you welcome each guest individually, dividing your time equally among them. Also, make sure the food items-snacks, drinks and sweets reach at each table and waiters' service at each table is quite right.

Don't forget to introduce your family members to the guests if they are unfamiliar to them. The oldest female member of the family should be introduced first. Make sure, guests never pass any unfavourable remarks on other guests. After the party, it is better if the host sends the "thank you" cards to the invitees.

Guests' Entertainment

Entertainment in the party is paramount. Let your family, relatives and friends join with one another in a funny, pleasant and relaxed atmosphere of the party. For this, you- as a host- can organize an outdoor sporting event such as badminton, volleyball or table tennis or any musical sport game etc. This will give the guests a perfect opportunity to interact with one another. Introduce the guests with one another by knowing their possible common interests. Encourage them to mingle with one another to make the party a grand success.

Novel Method to Charm Guests

Mrs. Shashi Mukherjee of Hazaribag suggests a new method to make the party an amusing event. She says that if it's a wedding party, couple can display their love story in writing, in a funny way on posters- how they met, how dotingly they talked; who proposed first, which movies they watched together and by fixing the writings in a frame they can display them for the guests to read. Let the guests enjoy the romantic moments. Pre-wedding video clips can also be showed on LED sets.

The collection of other photographs of the couple when they were kids and naughty can also be displayed on the poster board at party site. A family tree displaying the posterity of both the families can also be displayed.

Ashwini Ahuja

Ms. Rajni Wadhwa, a beautician says that party is the time to enjoy; you can discover several novel methods to enhance your happiness and the entertainment of your guests as well.

Hire a professional caterer

Taste attracts guests. Be sure about the preparation and provision of the delectable food items. For menu ideas and preparation, the service of professional caterer is the best option. Make sure if the desserts are tasty and drinks are branded. If not, guests will begin to hurl unfavourable comments over the arrangement of the party.

Professional caterer always advises their host to buy bulk of kitchen items so; do follow their guidelines. Hire the waiters/waitresses who are well dressed and groomed. They must be humble and soft speaking guys and gals also.

Decorated cakes with chocolate flavour are most liked items. Most ladies and the kids love to relish the cake pie. It must be served plentifully in pretty, colourful plates with coffee along with several types of sandwiches, pastries and sweetmeats.

In Tight Budget

Sometimes, the host of the party, in tight budget condition, prefers to buy cheap qualities food items and avoids quality decoration. It can mess up the grace of the party and annoys the guests as well.

Mr. Rajeev Makkar opines, in such economics, the host can pursue the creative ideas of decoration such as he/she can decorate the party venue with the photo collages including their childhood photographs. This way, they can both save the money and also give the party a fresh look.

Moreover, host can assigns the duty of photographing and video recording of the event to some of their reliable, expert & amateur family friends. Apart from it, inexpensive decorations such as heart-shaped balloons, red table clothes with the pictures of hearts can also be used for decoration. Heart shaped chocolate and candies can be distributed during musical games. On the party heart-shaped cake, the photos of the couple or family members with their names can also be decorated. Moreover, in tight budget, you need not buying fancy invitation cards.

Music Party

Music is the soul of every party. It enhances the beauty of the function and encourages the guests to tune up. If the host is planning to organize a big party then jazz band or mariachi band or both plus violin, acoustic guitar are perfect source of musical management.

If the budget doesn't allow hiring such arrangements then simple music, DJ and party dance by family women and friends can add charm and style to the party. But don't forget to make the music a part of the celebration.

Suggestions for Host

1 Don't make the party a nerve-racking and hectic situation. It must be a joyous time for all-friends, guests and the families.

Ashwini Ahuja

2 Don't invite anybody who you consider is not comfortable with other guests. If someone unexpectedly comes, accommodate him/her in a graceful and elegant manner. Don't speak rudely to him/her despite he/she uses coarse language for you to some extent.

3 To give the party a charm and style, you must include some persons who are good conversationalists and amuse a handful of people. Laughter kings are the heroes of any party.

4 For guests who live at distant places, firstly, invite them telephonically telling them about the reason of the party with date and time and then ask for their confirmation in the party.

5 If you are including the drinks in party, make sure the drink session should be concluded in time before dinner and you need not be extravagant in purchasing the drinks.

6 Open the gifts pack after the guests departed.

7 Don't forget, party is good time to relax and meet everyone. So, be calmed and free of anxiety. Display of strains onto your temple can upset the guests.

8 Meet everyone personally so as none feel ignored by you in the party.

9 Avoid talking on personal issues that may exclude other guests.

10 If you arrange the party at home, you must ensure there would be enough parking-space available for the guests.

Etiquettes for Guests

- When you are accepting the invitation, reply it quickly before inquiring who else is coming to the party.
- In party, if you are taking drink, don't binge on extravagantly.
- Come to the party with gifts but don't open the pack before the guests and don't let them know what you are giving them. They will know themselves, when they open the pack.
- If you have received the invitation and are unable to attend the party, must ring up and seek apology.
- Arriving late at the party is not a decent gesture, so arrive well in time.
- If some guests are staying with you, don't take them along to the party without knowing your host in advance.
- Be generous in thanking to the hosts.
- Must give compliments on their arrangements and choice of dishes etc.

Dinning Etiquettes

It is not only the hosts but the guests also should maintain the decorum of any party. If you are guests, be conscious regarding these points.

Ashwini Ahuja

1. Don't smoke at the table where you are eating with female guests.
2. As the lady approaches the dinning table to greet you, you too stand up to give her respect and sit down when she goes or sits down with you.
3. If you are sipping tea, don't dip biscuits into the cup and eat them foolishly.
4. While you visit another table to see the guests or friends, don't' pull the chair from other table without soliciting the persons who is sitting near it.
5. Don't rub your genitals while eating or when a lady friend or guest is sitting with you.
6. Don't put fingers into your nostrils.
7. Don't use tooth pick on dinning table if something gets struck in your teeth while you are eating.
8. Don't eat cake with a tea spoon and don't suck on fingers when it is finished.
9. Avoid the noise of your spoon when you are eating something.

Chapter Ten

PLASTIC USE IN KITCHEN

Plastic plays a vital role in our daily routine life. The markets all around the world are flooded with plastic bags, containers, utensils etc. It might not be exaggeration if one says life without plastic these days is quite impossible. Be its use in the kitchen or grocery stores, plastic largely dominates in every sphere of life.

Plastics are not just a means to place goods or articles in them. They are also used for commercial effects. Big showrooms and super markets also show their advertisements on them. Customers then become roaming publicity as they exhibit wherever they brought the goods in plastic bags at home.

An Inescapable Necessity

At grocery stores, plastic is used in the form of bags and containers for carrying several articles. In kitchen, it is used up in cups, plates, containers, tumblers, bowls and microwave wares etc. Plastic industry is booming day by day. No doubt, it is our inescapable

Ashwini Ahuja

necessity but have you ever thought about the safety of your health while using plastic in your daily life?

Plastic is more unsafe when we tend to use it beyond its original purpose. Most women at home store mineral water bottles for several months or until they break up. Don't forget they are meant for single use only. Sometimes, in our families, we carelessly use cheap, coloured plastic bags for packing hot food. Both situations are quite harmful.

If we follow the guidelines, mentioned on the products, we can guard ourselves from the vulnerability of the plastic. We should always keep in mind the utility, durability and dumping of the plastic products and moreover, temperature at which the particular types can be placed or used. Pouring the boiling food into ordinary heat-resistant plastic utensil can spoil the taste of the food

Food becoming dangerous poison

At the time of producing plastic products, different chemicals- styrene, phthalates & bisphenol are generally used.

When we use those plastic utensils inadvertently which are apparently not for that particular purpose in our daily life, the harmful chemicals are seeped into our food and we consume them with our food or drinks.

Even plastic bottles are more exposed to the heat of sun-light and high temperatures can lead to the exodus of dangerous chemicals into the water. So, never forget to discard the mineral water bottle after its first single use.

The quantities of seeping chemicals mostly depend on the nature and temperature of the food and longevity of contact time but overall, it is not a good practice for people seeking good healthy lifestyle.

Such chemicals in the human body dangerously affect the nervous system. Blood defects and carcinogenic effects can also be noticed as the signs of plastic hazards.

Take these precautions

1   Never use the plastic packaging repeatedly which is particularly designed for single use.

2   Never re-use the non-food packaging and containers; for example, detergents and washing soaps containers, for packing food items or lunch for school kids.

3   Don't put plastic containers inside microwave. Heat can dangerously leach chemicals into food.

4   Even so called microwave-safe plastic containers don't guarantee the release of chemical when they are over-heated.

5   So, always use ceramic, free of metallic paint or glass containers in microwave.

6   Never put disposable containers into microwave or into conventional oven as they are not heat-stable.

Ashwini Ahuja

7   Always use a paper towel, waxed paper or a plate for covering food.

8   Never think of cling wraps.

9   If there is nothing more than plastic wrap for covering the food items, be sure to keep the plastic wraps from touching the food items.

10   Ensure the maximum use of glass, glazed ceramic and stainless steel in kitchen.

11   Don't store pickles, jam and oily substances in ordinary plastic containers. These foods are more ready to absorb the plastic toxins into them.

12   If you don't get rid of all of your plastics anyway, at least discard old plastic containers, especially those that are profoundly worn out or scratched.

13   Older plastics are inclined to leach increasing amounts of toxins as they become old. Use them to store non-food items.

14   Generally, sliced cheese and meats are sold in tiny plastic bags and wraps; take them out as soon as possible and place them into a safe container or unbleached wax paper.

For Pregnant Women

Dr. Madhu Sharma, a gynaecologist says that the pregnant ladies particularly should be aware about the use of plastic in life. They should never forget BPA (Bisphenol A) chemicals will directly go to their babies through blood stream. They can harm the baby or cause the premature delivery.

Also, the other side effects of plastics are the lowering of sperms and early start of puberty. To defend ourselves from these health hazards, the option of bio-plastics is much better than the traditional plastics.

Dr. Madhu Sharma further says that bio-plastics are derived from vegetable oil, pea starch, shrub and corn starch etc., so it is not a bit harmful while traditional plastics which are derived from petroleum can give big loss to the healthy body.

Today, the markets are flooded with bio-plastic products like cups, water bottles, cutlery- forks, spoons, knives and containers etc. It is much better if pregnant ladies buy these eco-friendly products from markets for the welfare of their health, she concludes.

Combination of PVC & Phthalates

Nagpur based Dr. Ravindra Lavania says that PVC (poly vinyl chloride) and phthalates give much damage to the body. Plastics are the combination of these two substances. With these two substances, plastics become softer and pliable. In baby bottles, nipples, drinking water bottles and in storage containers, generally these substances are used. Moreover, most of the kitchen items are made of phthalates.

Ashwini Ahuja

Normally, in human bodies, phthalates are found which are known as destructive contaminants. These contaminants leach into body through plastic products & give them harm.

In Old Days

Dr. Lavania further says that in old days, people used to carry their baskets or cotton handbags while go for shopping in the markets. They gathered the all shopping items into their baskets or bags but now the time has drastically changed.

These days, for every item; plastic bags are recklessly used. They are everywhere either in the form of Tupperware or plastic wraps.

They are terribly bio-hazard as they are made from a variety of toxic chemicals. Plastic contaminates both our food and environment. At present, to get rid of the plastics in life is our main problem. Plastics are neither properly recycled nor they become destroyable within a rational length of time. If they are burnt, greenhouse gases are increased which pollutes the air. If we bury them, both the ground water and the soil pollute.

Encourage environment friendly substitute

Cathy Cirko, social activist associated with Canadian Plastics Association suggests it is much better if we encourage the trend of paper bags in our daily routine life.

No doubt, paper packets cost much more than plastic bags but these are environment friendly. The customers should be encouraged to take their own baskets or cotton bags when they go for shopping like in the old days.

Do efforts collectively

It must be ensured that a great deal of plastic never gets recycled. It must be a collective effort of both the shopkeepers and the customers to get rid of the anti-environment plastic hazards. Why don't we, first of all, think of making the disappearance of plastic bags from shopping complex?

If we remain careless for a long time regarding the use of plastics in our daily routine life, none might stop us becoming the victim of its cruel hazards.

Ashwini Ahuja

Chapter Eleven

SECURE SHOPPING FOR LADIES

Ladies! We know shopping is a passion for you. If there is one thing in the world that allures you most, it is the only shopping. Every lady prefers to go for it whenever she grabs the opportunity. Whenever she hears that there is a new mall opening or a sale bazaar in any part of the city, she picks her shopping bag and rush to that place.

And, in the shopping area, none can stop her to buy some articles of clothing, jewellery, cosmetics or fashion items etc. either she really requires these items or not but shopping is a necessity for her.

If you are also one of such ladies, be careful while moving about alone for shopping.

LADIES ARE SOFT TARGETS

Ladies having a purse filled with cash or other handy items are generally soft targets of street urchins or louts loitering around the markets.

If you are going for shopping late evening or night, be sure; you have a male companion with you. He may be your husband, relative, classmate, colleague or any other to whom you trust.

In most cases, before going for shopping avenue, ladies prefer to go to ATM for some cash in hand because every shopkeeper doesn't accept credit cards.

If you are inside the cabin for cash collect, be watchful about the surrounding. Observe if someone is eyeing on you in secret.

If it is so, be more alert and cautious. The people standing outside the ATM cabin know well that anyone coming out of the ATM is carrying cash.

And ladies are naturally soft targets because they are unable to hit back or thrash the ruffians like males if someone dares to snatch the cash from them. If it's early morning or the late night or evening, street urchins find place near the cabin or corridors for their sleep and it is not easy to ask them to leave the place.

If you are alone and planning to go for shopping, it would be better for you to go during busy hours. Early morning and late night, both are riskier for an alone lady.

CHOOSE A STRONG BAG WITH ZIPPERS

Handbag is a necessary item for the ladies who are moving out for shopping. In their handbags, ladies generally hold several important things such as credit cards, debit cards, driving license, mobile phone, cubboard keys, passport, UDI card, bank pass book, cheque book etc.

If your handbag is lost or torn down while you scuffle with a sort of urchin who is trying to snatch your bag from you, you will experience a serious trouble. So, to avoid the danger of any type, choose a strong zipper bag of good quality leather. Value your shopping bag a prized possession.

In another case, if your shopping bag fell down while you are scuffling with the urchins, if the zip of your bag is strong, things will not spill out. Always buy a shopping bag with loops so as it may slip through your arms.

This way you are able to snuggle the handbag under your arms tightly and securely and make your shopping safe and sound.

BE QUICK IN EVERY ACTIVITIES

If it is the dark evening or night and you are alone and standing in the mall for shopping. First thing; speak to the shop owner to send someone to carry the items, you have purchased, to the car.

Second thing, move briskly, the key to the car in your hand. It is the bad habit if someone lady stands near the car and zips open the shopping bag to fumble about the key inside the pocket of the purse. In this way, you will not mind on your personal safety and allow the predators to attack on you.

Alert! It is the riskiest moment when you may be the target of that urchin who is waiting for you next to your car. If there are a number of people moving around your car, be extra alert and act wisely.

If there is a guard or a policeman around there, don't hesitate to seek his help if necessary. After placing your items inside the car, don't wait for stay outside for any phone call or any kind of another triviality.

Generally, the ladies have a tendency for eating, drinking water or fumbling their purse after entering into the car but you don't do such trivial things. Start your car and lock its doors. Move it immediately. It is also a wrong habit if you begin to fumble about music system or begin to call to anyone over your cell phone or reading the SMSs.

It is no time for such types of unimportant things. Do you know who is watching you? Just move off the car. A moving car is rarely a target. Don't let the intruder an opportunity to break in your car and kidnap you. Some intruders are so much quick and act swiftly that general public fail to notice their transgression.

AVOID UNWANTED IDENTITY DOCUMENTS

No doubt, ID proof is an essential document one should have with him or her while going for outing. If you are going for outdoor shopping, you should also have any document of your ID proof with you.

Some ladies possess several documents such as PAN card, credit card, driving license, passport, office card or election card as their ID proofs in their purse. It is quite unnecessary to carry all these documents every day.

Ashwini Ahuja

What is the purpose of carrying so many important documents with you for all the time? Undoubtedly, you will keep these documents in your purse or handbag.

In case, your handbag is stolen or snatched by any street urchin or lout during shopping, what would happen, what you will do except for experience a series of trouble for next several months? Registration certificate of your vehicle is sufficient for your identity at that time. So, always be safe and secure and don't carry valuable documents with you except the one ID proof and that should be your driving license.

Moreover, ladies generally keep their cell phone in their handbags. If your handbag is snatched or stolen, your cell phone is also gone. And, you know, what is the meaning of losing cell phone when you are alone in shopping complex? You will be quite handicap without cell phone and can't even call for help.

So, ladies! Reduce your weight and get rid of unneeded and unnecessary articles for your safety and security.

DON'T CARRY EXPENSIVE JEWELERY

Diamond jewelry is very expensive items. Most ladies carry it in their purse whenever they go for shopping. Some wear it to show off their diamonds.

If you are going for shopping, you must not wear it as it may attract the attention of many street urchins on your way. Keep your ornaments in a box or a bag especially designed for them at home or bank locker and wear them on special occasion.

So, never carry your costly jewellery with you when you are travelling to the market for shopping whether there are security arrangements. Market is such a place where you may come across a lot of strangers in police uniforms also. And you may also be cheated or plundered by such scoundrels.

Unfortunately, if you lose it or someone snatches your jewellery from you, you will feel as if you have lost a part of your soul.

If you are wearing costly jewellery, the chances of attacks on you will be higher than a lady without wearing jewellery.

FINAL MESSAGE

Ladies! Let me deliver a final message for you. Shopping is not a bad thing after all. Make it a pleasant experience for you. Don't make it nightmarish experience and trouble your hubby and family.

ACT WISELY AND BE ON THE ALERT

If someone breaks in your car just after you are stepping into it after shopping. Don't be afraid. It is the time for you to attract the attention of others. You may attract the attention of others by flashing the lights of your car or blowing the horn aggressively. Try your best to lower the window and cry for help. Loud voice of female drivers catches the attention of others quickly. Then you see wonders! People will run towards you to defend you.

If you are alone while going for shopping, take elevator instead of stairwells as most of the crimes and the incidents of plundering are happened there

Some women suggest an umbrella, an object for their safety. You can also carry it when you go for shopping as it can be used as a weapon from a distance.

Never try to be sympathetic in the market when you are alone. You may come across a serial killer like the Ted Bundy who played the sympathies of unsuspecting women by walking limp and seeking help into his car. Then he abducted the woman and raped her.

Never put on scintillating or scanty dresses while go for shopping. Showing off too much flesh invites unnecessary risk. Avoid eye contact with unwanted male loitering in the market. If you are paying cash to any shopkeeper, don't take out more money out of the purse than it is necessary for payment.

Chapter Twelve

Enhance Your Face Value

Do you know the value of smiling face? Increasing stress, anxiety and unbendable pressure have preoccupied our minds hauntingly. And these days, we have completely forgotten to smile even a little.

In our offices or working places, we meet our colleagues and friends casually wearing worries on our faces. Such unworthy attitude weakens our ties with colleagues and hampers the pace of our work in office.

It is quite true, these days, down to ambitions; we are deadly busy in our homes as well as at our workplaces but it doesn't mean that we should forget to express our happiness through smiling faces while we come across friends and colleagues.

Remember, smiling is such a finest facial expression that denotes pleasure and happiness. The more we meet others with smiling face, the more we command respect and love from others.

Smile, sure enough, is the beginning of the love and the pleasant emotions and moreover, it frees us from strain and worries.

Sociologist's Opinions

Sociologist Alok Sharma says that through smiles, one can communicate emotions. He says that smile shows that how much happy we are.
Money is not everything. One can earn enough money by hard working but smile is more difficult to earn than money if it is lost. So, never lose it, come what may.

Alok Sharma further says that smiling is a simplest, easiest and cheapest ever way to build a connection among people as well as improve our looks and even moods.

It is a like a bridge between two hearts. When we frown, forty three muscles of our face have to work but if we are smiling, only seventeen muscles work to spread smiles so what is the purpose of wasting our energy by frowning.

When someone smiles, brain releases endorphins which make us feel happy and better.

Positive Attitude Brings Smile

If your attitude is quite positive, there is no reason you will not be happy and in high spirits. One can't define happiness easily just in a few words. It is essentially a state of mind where we are completely satisfied with ourselves.

In offices, we generally ignore our colleagues and friends due to competitive jealously. We don't meet them happily and don't smile to know about their achievements. Remember, if you smile for sometimes, you must forget your worries and anxieties.

Imagine, how a smiling child looks beautiful and sweet? Everybody loves to play with a cute smiling face child.

Dr. Vinod Sharma, a career strategist says that in a competitive life of today, it is much difficult to be happy in life but if you are happy and ever smiling face, you are blessed one.

Simple point is: if your attitude is positive, you will be happy and your face always will be smiling. The art of happiness can only be achieved with positive attitude. If you are pessimistic and have a negative attitude, neither you can smile nor win in the face of harsh conditions.

Contentment Multiplies Smile

Ashwini Ahuja

Think; you are contented with yourself? If not, first of all you need to be contented with yourself. Then, it might be easy for you to smile unreservedly because contentment multiplies smile and happiness. Don't forget to smile even in your bad times.

No matter, you have bank balance in millions or every means of luxury also but if you are not contented with yourself, you will not be able to smile.

Help Others and Be Happy

If you help others in the times of their need, you will bring smile not only on your faces but put a smile on other's faces also. Prof. M. S. Verma says that by helping elders and treating everyone equally creates a positive impact on others and you can make them smile with your helping hands.
Smile is contagious. It is such a great thing which can be done as a part of our normal routine and cost nothing. By helping others with smiling face, you will be surprised to see how many people are encouraged by your kindness.

So, don't let insatiability and self-interest rule your heart ever. Always meet everyone with smile because it is the only smile which begins love.

Brings smile on Others' Face

Give someone an inspiration book to read and then see how miraculously you have brought smile on his/her face. When he/she reads the book, he/she will think of you. Write a hand written encouraging note for someone to give him/her inspiration and show him/her or send him/her by post. You will see a permanent smile on his/her face when you see him/her.

Deliver a meal or tea to someone at the time of their need when he is sick and at bed rest. When he comes out of the bed, he will always greet you with beauteous smile. Don't forget to thank anyone who helps you at your request or at the time of your need to view smile on his face in future.

Always reveal a genuine smile to everyone you meet then you will see how easy it is to get others to smile.

Thirteen Chapter

Social Twittering

These days, twittering on social networking sites is a fad among teens. Oxford University study says that social networking has bad effects on kids' brainpower and damage could be long lasting and irrevocable. On the other side, the aficionados of social networking sites defend that teens and kids are doing better than adults while increasing their social interaction with friends and wiring their brains to adapt to new technology.

At the present time, social networking sites especially for kids and teens have become an inescapable part of their life. Grown ups, professionals and socialite ladies too use social networking sites for communication, befriending and business deals etc. but for teens, these sites are their favourite haunts.

They interact with friends through these sites, share photographs, make new friends, fight, argue and share their routine and family problems etc also. They prefer these sites for chatting with friends than connecting with friends in real life.

A Good Medium for Social Contact

The question is: a virtual social world is the right place for communication? Our relations with real friends, neighbours, relatives and close family members are shrinking day by day.

In such a situation, social networking world is more important than the real world? Moreover, is it a good medium for real friendships, business deal, exchange photographs, love and long lasting relationships, for dating, love chat, fighting, arguing without meeting the people face to face and in flesh and blood.

Varun Gagneja, a forensic expert says that social networking sites especially the face book is a wonderful place for meeting friends. I have made a lot of friends through this site. Also, I have learnt a lot of unknown things about my friends through this medium. I have been able to showcase my photography talents to the large audience only due to facebook.

Varun Gagneja further warns that parents of the adolescents should be alert. They should not allow their children and teens to eat into the real relationship time.

Several reports on social media also say that the children and adolescents are spending a lot of time on social networking sites. These sites have created a lot of impact on them.

Varun says that these sites offer both risks and benefits to teens. For an introvert, these sites are a godsend giving them the opportunities to socialize but for an extrovert commoner, they are quite unsafe.

Come what may, Varun Gagneja concludes that the excess use of social twittering with friends on networking sites has eaten into our direct contact by taking us away from real friends, relatives and colleagues and it's the worst effect of social networking sites on us.

A Fad More Than a Necessity

Ms. Swati Shrivasta, an executive at Dabur India, Delhi says that in India, social networking is a fad more than a necessity but it is good for reclusive and introvert folks to engage in socially without meeting face to face as the virtual space is performing incognito.

Swati further says that the best part of this fad is that it has made our youths creative and innovative. Our generation is now honing their composition skills through fascinating and informative blogs in spite of old technique of essay writing or paragraphing notes.

Needless to say that blogging on social networking sites or writing notes on facebook sites have generated numerous writers and readers as well. It is almost a good trend.

Although the trend of reading books has replaced reading on networking sites or reading the blogs but it's not our necessity for the life. It is a just a fad which we think it is our necessity and the day we don't

---

Ashwini Ahuja

log on facebook or any other social networking site, we think that we have lost something that day.

Do More Harm Than Good?

According to reports on the importance of social media, more than 150 million people log on facebook every week to keep in touch with friends, relatives, colleagues and others and share photographs and videos etc. On twitter, more than six millions people have signed up. They too share their news to thousands. Undoubtedly, these sites are much popular and are beneficial to all of us. But a number of neuroscientists and psychologists opine that these sites are doing more harm than good. These sites encourage instant gratification, shorten attention spans and make our teens and young people self centred and egotistical.

The excess use of social networking sites have made our youngsters the victims of insomnia as they are reported to be hooked on these sites all through the night.

Prof MS Verma says that overall, social networking sites are good but when they are misused and abused, several big problems arise.

When one becomes dependent on social networking sites, they ruin their personal and family life. Moreover, the exposure to audio visual and social networking sites throughout their adolescence makes them disillusioned and sceptical by the time they attain adulthood.

The common problem with facebook is: kids and teens are not aware of the posts they put on others' wall.

Sometimes, negative wall posts cause them anxiety and tension.

A Safe Zone for Shy People

It is said that social networking sites are a safe zone for those who are shy and slow in their real life. On these sites, such people feel safer to initiate conversations. It is less threatening and more comfortable for people who are otherwise fearful of having direct, head-on conversations with others. Often, people use these sites as a platform to make important announcements and inform each others about their new businesses and individual's developments in their life.

Through these sites, the users can get instant reactions of their assignments or pieces of writings if they post on these sites.

Parents' Supervision is required

A housewife Mamta Jain says that all social networking sites have an age criteria where one should be at least eighteen years of age to create an account. But unfortunately, we notice that children even below ten years of age are accessing their facebook, orkut or other social networking accounts.

In such cases, much attention ought to be paid to secure the account of children. It is more important for parents to supervise the activities of their children on social networking sites and make the site's privacy secure.

Parents should further be aware about the mental and emotional maturity level of their children and keep in mind that their youngsters may not get exposed to inappropriate information or material. They should never be extremely addictive to these sites, anyway.

It is the time when our young minds should be engaged in dealing with the realities of life and relationships and they should not be allowed dipping their body and souls into a virtual reality.

Mamta further says that at this time, the youngsters are generally more prone to being addicted to social networking sites. Years back, the same people were gripped with comic books and video games. Now, the habits have replaced with interaction with friends on social networking sites and playing online games on internet.

Journalist Nisha Verma opines that most social media sites are good and helping kids in several ways. It is the only social networking sites where children socialise and connect together but the supervision of the parents is essential.

She suggests that the parents should be friends with their children on facebook or any other site. If the child don't want his parents a friend, it is the clear sign that something is happening wrong with him or her.

In such a situation, don't allow to sit your child on computer while he/she is wishing to log on social networking sites. In general life, parents don't allow their children to drive a car alone without learning them, in the similar way, social networking is also risky.

Don't assume that your kid knows the all things. Kids and teens must be thoroughly taught that how facebook works. Doing such thing is necessary for protection of child from online predators and other dangers.

Always advise your child to take advantage of social networking to enhance learning. Teach them the difference between the substance and the trash. Don't forget to warn your kid while he is trying to engage himself in the darker side of the social networking like cyber bullying, sharing inappropriate materials etc.

Essential for Success

About talking over the pros and cons of the social networking sites, Ms Mamta Jain says that today is the age of internet. These days, we all depend on internet for everything.

Internet is used for shopping and marketing, bank transaction, railway and air reservation, paying telephone and electricity bills and meets others and also to find what we are looking for. For business deals, internet is the fastest way. Thus, without being social conversation, it is hard to run business in a good way.

So, needless to say that social networking is essential for success. Through these sites, we not only make friends but make business contacts also. These contacts impact our future success with an online business.

Moreover, social networking sites are used for social or political cause also. These days, several politicians are using social media to garner votes and support from their voters, workers and well wishers etc. What

Ashwini Ahuja

is more, even marriages are also fixed on social networking sites.

If we look back, in 2001, a social activist Ajay Kumar of Mumbai had started a campaign on Twitter for cancer patients and collected around Rs: twenty lakhs within a short span of time.

During his last election, Barack Obama too contacted millions of people on a very personal level with the help of Twitter. And after that Anna Hazare's fight against corruption too is noticed on several social networking sites.

Doctor's Opinion

Dr. Amit Sachdeva says that social networking sites make the kids self centred. They affect kids' comprehension level. While communicating through the screen, kids don't learn the subtleties of real life communication such as body language, tone of voice etc.

Dr. Amit further says that today, we observe several teens suffering from facebook depression. The teenagers who spend most of their time on social networking sites become moody and anxious.

Facebook and other social networking sites provide kids their own page which is all about them. Sensitive teens think that everything revolves around them. It is a clear sign for emotional problems of children in the later stage of their life.

Dr. Anju Setia opines that social networking sites make the kids prone to sensationalism. Moreover, social networking sites' kids are weaker in spelling and grammar than all those students who rarely log on any social networking site. Throughout their life, communication with misspellings and lack of grammar are seeping through their school's writings.

Contrary to it, Mac Arthur Foundation, America claims that kids and teens are developing significant technical and social skills online in a ways that adults don't even understand. So, spending time online is necessary for young people to know the social and technical skills in this digital age.

Through social networking, for kids and teens, it has become easier to make friends with people all over the world, most of whom they will never meet without these sites and get a chance to talk to them due to time and cost restraints. These sites also make kids relationship oriented and emphatic. They remember friends' birthday and greet them.

In a nutshell, we can say that social networking sites are more good than bad for teens if we manage their depression and always supervising their activities on social networking sites.

Ashwini Ahuja

Chapter Fourteen

Tattoo Artist: Enjoy the Passion

These days, the trend of tattoos is at the height of fashion. Tattoos are considered the latest things to delight the mood of our youngsters, kid, socialite and the sophisticated ladies of the modern society.

In old times, no well-brought-up person would love sporting tattoos on their skin but today, not only the common fashionable guys and ladies but even the military personnel and other different cultural and tribal groups have also started sporting tattoos on their bodies.

Some ladies have passion for tattooing. If you are such lady, you may enjoy the passion by choosing a career as tattoo artist. The demand for an expert tattoo artist is soaring. So, by becoming a good tattoo artist, you may make good money in this profession

The job of a tattoo designer or artist is to design and create a lifelike picture to be permanently tattooed on a customer's body

Obviously, there is a trend of sporting ankle or wrist tattoos among college girls, models and film stars so as they look smart and stylish and quite different from others. These two areas- ankle and wrist- are considered the best places by them to get tattoos done because these areas always remain slim during the most of their life. Needless to say that tattoos are very fashionable today among all generations.

In old days, tattoos were not reputable and tattooing could not be a viable profession. It was not accepted by society wholeheartedly. That time, tattoos were sported by only low-life bikers, goons and drug addicts, but that was not the era of cable television. But, now, the modern technology has changed people's way of thinking.

So, the negative connotation which had been in the past has now completely changed and tattooing has become a style statement. It is, at present, a profitable and good business. What to say, athletes too began to sport several tattoos covering the ninety percent of their bodies.

Become an Expert Tattoo Artist

As the demand for tattoo artist is frequently soaring. So, there are several aspirants opting to join in tattoo business. Practice makes the man perfect.

Ashwini Ahuja

Apart from educational qualification for this profession, you need to have as much as necessary practice to become a successful tattoo artist or a designer. Don't forget that a practical internship is the best way to learn the art of tattooing.

A successful tattooist can make money-spinning living applying tattoos on the bodies of his customers. But, always remember that this job is not quite easy and simple.
Rajni Wadhwa, a beautician says that it is not like something that you wake up in the morning and decide to set up a tattoo studio.

It takes skill and deep knowledge of the subject and moreover the artistic bent of mind.

For lazy, slothful and non-creative aspirants, tattoos artistry is not a good career at all. If you dream to be a successful designer in tattoo industry, you need to be artistic, self-driven and always dedicated.

Dr. Anju Sachdeva opines that the first basic step to become the tattoo artist is: you must have developed some creative talent in you such as the ability to draw and colour within lines and for that practice, you also must have a mentor. Without having a guru, it is not possible for you to develop requisite skills.

If you think that without studying various art and design books and without a practice for long time, just watching the other people doing the work, you can become the expert tattoo artist; it is not possible for you. To earn the accomplishment, practice is important. You should create a portfolio of your best designs or artworks to show the prospective clients or your employers to get a good job of tattoo artist in tattoo industry.

Keep Yourself Updated

If you think that you have practised for a short time and you become an expert and you can earn thousands a day, you are wrong. Practice for a short period doesn't yield good result.

Tattoo artistry demands that you must keep your mind open to new ideas forever. For updates, you should visit the different places to view the tattoos shows in different exhibitions that are organized by the big tattoos studios.

Like any other profession, in tattoo business, customers expect the best quality, health care and service from tattoos artists also.

So, it is also very important to listen to your clients and make sure what exact artwork they desire to create on their bodies. It is much difficult for you to create a real life image what your client expect from you if you are without updates and new ideas.

Ashwini Ahuja

Only by being proficient and with updates, you will be able to satisfy your clients. Don't be wild when you have a plentiful customers, you must consult with your every client about the designs, shape, colours and the placement of the tattoos they are interested in. Never be rude and unethical to your customers. Being rude is not a good sign for a good business.

Sterilization and Sanitation

Hygiene is very important issue in the case of tattooing. A tattoo artist or a designer is required to abide the rules, policies and guidelines set by the health ministry regarding the sterilization and sanitation to avoid spreading blood borne diseases like HIV/AIDS or hepatitis.

So, keep updated yourself with up-to-the-minute changes in the rules and policies of the government to cover the health risk of not only of your clients but your own risk also if it arises in any condition.

Doctors generally advise every tattoo artist to use disposable syringes or sterilized ones for each customer to prevent blood borne diseases and they should be obeyed as ditto.

Next point: a tattoo artist should never forget to scrub tubes before placing them in an ultrasonic and also never forget to sterilize them in an autoclave. Doing so must be a daily process for a tattoo artist. One time use products such as razors and ink caps are also necessary for a safe environment.

It is very essential to spray down workstations, chairs and other equipments with a germicidal spray before and after each tattoo for safety.

In sporting the tattoos, the ink is applied to the base layer of the skin. If the tattoo designer applies the ink to the top layer of the skin, the image doesn't last long as the top layer is constantly renewing itself. So, it is the prime duty of the tattoo artist to tell the customers how they can properly care for their tattoos.

Education is required

The positive point in tattoo learning is that this art can be learned without having formal education in any college but it does not mean that you need not any training or intensive study of the subject.
Renowned tattoo artists suggest that one of the best ways to start an education as a tattoo artist is to contact an approved tattoo studio and get apprenticeship.

That apprenticeship may last for two to three years or more depending upon the talents and the time the aspirants devote for this profession.

To become a tattoo artist, some aspirants choose to obtain an art degree. It is better to become a skilled tattoo artist but if you are unable to get formal education, an apprenticeship from a studio will be sufficient for you becoming an expert in tattooing. But be sure, you have a license for this task.

Ashwini Ahuja

Apprenticeship will teach you the understanding of forms and colour technology. If you are good at drawing, you will learn the art of tattooing in a shorter period otherwise you will have to practice drawing a lot of original, beautiful and unique designs.

After training or apprenticeship, you need to prepare your portfolio. Always remember that it is your portfolio that will establish that you have the skills needed to succeed in the industry. To become an expert tattoo artist, you will have to learn the history of tattoo art, drawing, painting, illustrations and other forms of visual art apart from methodology and various specialized skills also.

No doubt, in some colleges, aspiring students hone their skills but it is not a requirement for being a successful in the art of tattooing.

Remember that formal training is certainly not the only way to make you expert. Informal practice or learning may develop you a prolific tattoo designer.

Rajni Wadhwa, a beautician says that without being diligent in practicing, there is no scope for a successful career in this field. Practice is more important than any college class for someone who is dedicated and able to develop his talents.

Conclusion

Moreover, it is vitally important to understand that tattoo artists have more responsibilities than simply applying a piece of permanent artwork to a client's leg, arm or back.

Education, safety, hard practice and training are most important components in the daily job requirements of a tattoo artist.

Last but not least: be creative, hard worker, keen observer and practical to see your career of tattooing flourishing day by day!

Points to Remember

If you desire to become an expert tattooist

- ✓ Learn the art of producing a variety of styles
- ✓ Learn new concepts and techniques
- ✓ Keep your interest in visual art and drawing intact
- ✓ Put your customers' health and safety above convenience
- ✓ Keep your equipments clean and sanitized
- ✓ Practice tattooing from each angle
- ✓ Study the intensive education as well as training from any approved tattoo studio
- ✓ Interact with your customers gently and friendly and offer best services to them
- ✓ Understand the basic anatomy and kinetics
- ✓ Be assertive when it is necessary

Chapter Fifteen

T-Shirts for Elegance and Style

Have you ever reflected, by wearing Tee-shirts, how much you look elegant, stylish and pleasing to the eyes? In summer, it is one of the most comfortable apparels for both men and women.

In recent times, it has become an acme of informality and qualities quotient. Moreover, it is convenient in rainy season as it needs not extensive washing plus short drying schedule. Be it sports events, swimming at pool or casual outing for dinner; T shirt serves as an all-purpose apparel.

T-Shirt: A wardrobe Staple

Typically, Tee-shirt or T-shirt, which can be dubbed as a wardrobe staple- is made of cotton with a mix of polyester fibers. It is a kind of cute shirt which is pulled on over the head to cover most of wearer's front particularly torso and it is also decorated with the pictures of celebrities and some odd texts as well.

World's largest companies too advertise their products through T- shirts. Its distinctive soft texture attracts the ladies and men of all age groups.

It is an enjoyable and relaxing experience to wear T-shirt while go for stroll.

Different Trends

Generally, T-shirt is apparel which extends slightly over the shoulder but not completely over the elbow. Either they are short or long, V-neck or round neck-its all variants are popular among youths and ladies. In its initial stage, T-shirts were worn as undershirts like the vests but today they are used as independent outfits.

Since the time of its origin, T-shirts which extend to waists are typically liked but in hip hop fashion, the craze of long T-shirts-which extended down to the knees, was developed.

In 1990, a trend of "tight-fitting-cropped" T- shirts among women came. That time women began to wear such T-shirts which were too short revealing their midriff.

Later, a trend of "layering" was also arrived when both men and ladies began to wear short sleeved T-shirt of a different colour over the long sleeved T-shirt.

Ashwini Ahuja

Cotton-Polyester Blend is Ideal

The majority of T-shirts are made of 100% cotton but T-shirts connoisseurs and buffs like to wear those T-shirts which are made of the mixture of polyester and cotton so as to get rid of the problem of shrinking. Purely cotton made T shirts generally shrink when they are first-washed but its cotton-polyester blend defeats the shrink problem.

T-Shirts for All Age Group

Markets are flooded with new styles and gracious designs for all - baby, youth and adults etc. In old times, T-shirts had been usually pocketless, buttonless and collarless but now it is available with different classy pockets and varieties of buttons.

Working women generally wear it for the protection from the sun. It has replaced their traditional outfit viz. saris, salwar kameez, traditional jumper etc.

Young collegiate- both boys and girls and office goers wear it for conviviality and fashion as it is more convenient to them especially while they are long travelling or working arduously in their offices.

Earlier, T-shirts were loved by kids and teens only. Now, it is liked and bought by the people of all age groups. These days, old age people prefer collared T-shirts and kids buy those T-shirts which are displaying several cartoon themes styles on them.

History Beckons

If we look back, it was the British Navy which firstly is said to have introduced the T-shirt. That time the sailors of British Navy used to wear sleeveless undershirts and their hairy armpits were nuisance to the royal officials during parades. They were advised to wear short sleeves to conceal the mess of their armpits. In the fifties, movie idols James Dean and Marlon Brando came up with new fashion when they combined the T-shirts with jeans. This fashion charmed the youths and a trend of wearing T shirt arrived.

In the early 1950, Miami based "Tropix Togs" was the first ever company which started decorating T-shirts with different resort names. Later, another Miami based organization "Sherry Manufacturing Company" came up with innovative styles & designs.

In 1959, a durable and stretchable ink namely plastisol was used to create much more varieties in T shirts designs. In 1960, a different type T-shirt which was known as ringer T-shirt appeared and became a staple fashion for youth and rock-n-rollers.

The Emergence of Fine Art Designs for T-shirts

In the same year also, Richard Ellman, Robert Tree, Stanley Mouse and others established a company namely "Monster Company" in California to create fine art designs for T-shirts.

A fashion designing course's student opines that T-shirt first became popular in America in twentieth century. In 1920, the word T-shirt or Tee-shirt with its meaning was included in Merriam-Webster's Dictionary.

Protection from Ultraviolet Rays

Ashwini Ahuja

No doubt, T-shirts are for all times but in summer season, this fabric is mostly loved by Indians. Exposure to sun's harmful rays infuriate several people who intend in enjoying outdoor activities. Firstly, Harvey Schakowsky, an American textile engineer had introduced a type of sun-blocking T-shirts which blocked out as most as 99 percent ultraviolet rays.

At present, such T-shirts are not common but typical T-shirt blocks out 50 percent of the rays. They are made out of synthetically woven cotton and nylon with the blending of chemical substance.

T-Shirts Signify Personality

You must have seen Sania Mirza, world's renowned tennis player wearing T shirts of different colours and different quotes display in the midst of the fabric such as "Attitude Unlimited" and "Well behaved women rarely make history" etc. What does it show?

Connoisseurs say that one's outfits speak one's personality. It displays the character and behaviour of the wearer also. The shirts with attitude slogans such as "God Bless You", "Flower Friend", "Think Green"; "Protect Yourself" are mostly liked by people. In 1980, in UK also, T- shirts with bold slogans were as popular as it never had been earlier.

T-Shirt: Corporate Trend of Dressing

In India, today, a new trend of wearing T shirt with corporate logo or slogan has emerged. Ladies working with "corporate world" love to wear short sleeve T-shirts contrasting bound neck band and cuffs. Among office going people, T-shirts with white, green, sky blue, navy, sunflower and olive colours are liked and worn tastefully.

Management experts say that wearing T-shirts while meeting with subordinate staff or co-workers gives a sense of affability and conviviality.

In the corporate world, T-shirts are preferably used to motivate employees as well as building brand loyalty in the market. The display of company's mottos and slogans on T-shirts show the attitude of the company and its employees.

Evolution of Style Modifications

At present, there are numerous style modifications in T-shirts which are available in the markets but a few are commonplace and liked by most of the fashion savvy.

Half Sleeve

Half sleeve cut T-shirts are good for summer season when scorching sun infuriates in its enormity. Such type stuffs are worn with both shorts and trousers as well. This type gives one's shoulder and chest more shape and meaning. Half sleeves are liked by all- kids, men and ladies.

Full Sleeve

Ashwini Ahuja

Since the seventies, full sleeve has been an accepted design by both men and women. It has multiple benefits. It protects the wearer's arm from getting tanned.

Moreover, if you have thin arms, full sleeve T-shirt can make them appear fuller. Contrary to it, if your arms are heavy, by choosing a dark colour full sleeve T-shirt, you can make your arms looking slimmer.

Cut sleeve

Cut sleeve T-shirts are good on thin as well muscular arms. To give an ideal look of an athlete to your body, it is a perfectly considerable option. Cut sleeve T-shirts give the wearer a casual and rough look.

Its both types- either it is the V-neck or the round-neck are ideal match for this cut. Cut sleeve is ideally good for comfort and ventilation. Fashion Designer Shruti Malhotra says that it is the "cut and fit" quotient in T-shirts which can radically change its look and style.

Round Neck T-shirt

Round Neck T-shirt is suitable for both men and ladies with long necks and slightly drooping shoulders as this style enwraps the base of neck on all sides. It is a casual dress for all recreational activities.

V-Neck T-Shirt

V-Neck is ideal for those having broad shoulders and thick neck. This cut gives the wearer a sporty and an athletic feel. It is shaped by two crosswise lines from the shoulder meeting on chest at a midpoint of T-shirt.

Apart from it- Tank Top, Muscle Shirt, Scoop Neck- some are other variations of T-shirts which are also liked by people.

Jeweled Design T-Shirts

Fashion Designer Shruti Malhotra says that in metros, the trend of jewelled designed and embroiled T-shirts is also hot.

Sometime ago, Kolkata based Mr. Shantanu, a student of National Institute of Fashion Technology, Kolkata had designed a kind of jewelled T-shirt with the theme of Lord Krishna's character.

That theme was most liked by textile companies and that brand was promoted globally. Shruti Malhotra further says that digital jewelled T- shirt bearing attitude themes are uniquely popular these days. Among young girls of metro cities, the trend of wearing T-shirt with mini skirts or jean pant is also ubiquitous.

Future of T-shirts Booming

T-shirts connoisseurs say that the future of the T-shirt industry in India is booming. Bollywood movies, film stars and celebrities play a significant role in promoting the brand of T-shirts.

Ashwini Ahuja

Sometimes, people are not aware of the new collection but when they see in films, actor/actress wearing T shirts, they buy the same brand for themselves. The time is not far away, Ms. Shruti Malhotra concludes, when we will see newer and innovative brands in the coming days. The future of the T-shirt is undoubtedly bright.

Chapter Sixteen

VELVET DRESS

Velvet has a long history. No wardrobe is complete without velvet. It is the favourite fabric of sophisticated ladies, models and cinema gals. Mothers too love to buy velvet clothes for their tiny, cute babies.

Whether, it is the fashion ramps or night parties, velvet is everywhere and it is awfully dominating the fashion world and hold your breaths, men also find the texture of velvet very tempting on women.

Ladies wearing velvet blouses are the attraction of men. They look richly affluent in exquisiteness and go well with both light and heavy sarees. You can wear saree with velvet borders or velvet designs and grab the attentions of the men you love or dream to have relationship with them

Winter season is the perfect time to wear velvet outfits. Whether it is the holiday parties or the family gathering, velvet is always unique and beyond compare. One can dress it with T-shirt- jeans or salwar kameez. Even it looks finely stylish with typical standard sarees.

Needless to say that it makes the looks of gents and ladies like tinsel super stars and queens. The markets at present are brimming with velvet products such as garments, accessories, lingerie, night dresses, hair accessories, handbag, footwear and shoes and moreover, jackets, blazers, cardigans with velvet lining inside that peeps out here and there which gives the ladies attractively sexy looks.

In winter, velvet outfits give the wearer the feelings of luxury and sensuality and warmth. Fashion designer Lalit Sharma says that velvet has deep and rich colours such as violet, purple, dark brown, olive green, blue and black etc.

Generally, velvet is chunky so, it is very essential that it would be well tailored to create its appearance some slim and dapper when you dress in.

Ashwini Ahuja

VELVET VS VELVETEEN

Fashion designers say that velvet and velveteen looks the same but actually it is not so. Velveteen is artificial velvet and it has less sheen. It is normally made of cotton or a combination of cotton and silk but velvet is made from silk, rayon, nylon, polyester etc. It has a very close and dense pile. Velvet is basically woven as a double cloth.

During the weaving process, the double cloth is separated. Moreover, velveteen doesn't drape easily and it is not as expensive as velvet. Velveteen makes the wearer look slimmer when wearing it than the wearing of velvet. Velveteen is easier to sew. It is also easy to launder. You can wash it at home also. It can also be dried in front of a radiator or gas fire also. Velvet is available in several kinds such as cotton, silk and satin but for dresses, silk is considered the best fabric. Fashion designer Lalit Sharma says that velveteen, velour and corduroy often looks like velvet but they are not actually comfortable, rich, soft, plushy and glossy like silk velvet clothing.

Always remember that velvet is woven traditionally using silk or even polyester while velveteen is made from cotton. Some people misconstrue the brasso a type of velvet. But, it is actually not so.

Although, there is a wide variety of imported velvet available in the markets but ladies in general love to wear Indian velvet as the Indian velvet has a two toned shadow effect that positively gives the outfits a vintage look. What is more, ladies love to dress flocking velvet- a sort of satin materials with velvet motifs embellished on it.

HOW TO WEAR VELVET

Ladies! All velvet and no other stuff is not a good fashion. Velvet always looks good with combinations and contrasts. To make your looks graceful, always try to wear velvet in small parts. If you have a medium or stout body build, you may wear velvet borders or small designs on your clothing. If you have a slim figure, you may wear full velvet clothes both on the upper and lower portion of your body. For slim figure, all velvet is quite fine. It will make your look slightly larger and charming.

For plump ladies, velvet on both portions of the body is not advisable as it will make the looks slightly larger and plumpness will expose more.

In winter, wearing velvet makes the look extremely chic, cool and sexy. Wearing velvet tunic with "tight and knee high boots" will make your looks attractive. If you love to wear top skirt, velvet tops definitely will give you the feelings of classiness.

Fashion Designer Lalit Sharma says as for the fine velvet dress, only velvet jacket or skirt is fine. Never dress the velvet pant and velvet jacket together. It won't look fine.

In brief, you should wear one piece of velvet at a time. Don't pair a velvet blouse with velvet saree or a velvet salwar with a velvet kameez or velvet shirt with pant. Doing overdo velvet is bad practice.

Lalit Sharma further says that velvet has its several plus points except for its rich fabric which adds sheen

Ashwini Ahuja

to the clothes. To give a fantastic and delicate feminine look to your appearance, you can try a velvet skirt with an antique sari border. One can give it fresh personalized look with embroidery or embossing if your velvet piece has worn out.

Lalit Sharma suggests that one should wear pristine and plush velvet to make your appearance beautiful but remember that don't wear the same colour velvet pant with velvet shirt.

COMPLIMENT YOUR VELVET OUTFIT

Fashion Designer Alka Goswami says that undoubtedly, velvet is a rich fabric. When you wear it, you should do a good amount of make-up to complement your outfit.

Generally, ladies prefer to highlight their eyes and lips with glossy lipsticks. If you have a common coloured velvet blouse, you can wear it with several sarees to give your style a few different statements. Although, velvet is always in vogue but it is practicable in cold climates. Alka Goswami says that it is actually a dress for winter season.

She further says that undoubtedly, a velvet outfit is a jewel in itself so when you wear velvet, don't over accessorize. Keep your jewelries simple. You may wear a chunky classic pendant in a gold chain and keep your ears, fingers and wrists bare. The buzz word is: enjoy flaunting your velvets.

Lalit Sharma says that velvet is the darling of winter but one may wear it throughout the year. It is formal as well as a dressy wear. Ladies may keep their velvet dresses and velvet skirts longer for formal parties whereas keep the shorter ones for cocktails and dinner parties.

Alka Goswami says that some models wear velvet salwar kameez in glitzy shows or performances but there is no match if we compare it with the charm of velvet sarees. In fact, salwar kameez with velvet borders or small designs look more graceful than full velvety kameez.

GOOD QUALITIES OF VELVET

- ✓ Velvet is warmer than silk. It is soft, luxurious, bright, flowing and radiant. Silk or silk viscose mixes are wonderful and they are apt for evening or night parties
- ✓ It is complimentary to all body types
- ✓ They drape well and good for evening wear also
- ✓ Children look smart and active and elegant in velvets

VELVET DIRECTIVES

1. If you are wearing a velvet dress. Don't carry a velvet handbag along with it.
2. No velvet accessories with velvet dresses. If you wear velvet jacket, make sure, there is no velvet clothing or accessory other than jacket.
3. Silk velvets are slippery to handle. It is more difficult to sew them than cotton velvets. So, be careful while you check in the tailor.

Ashwini Ahuja

4   Always remember that its fitting should be tailored well.

4   Velvet gives good result when it is dried cleaned. Don't press it in the normal way of pressing. To remove the wrinkles, turn it inside out. Use the velvet board if possible.

5   If velvet is stained, clean it with cold-water-dipped wet terrycloth

It is said that velvet wool was originated in Kashmir around the beginning of fourteenth century. During the regime of Harun Al Rashid, this fabric was introduced to Baghdad. It is said that in Mamluk era, Cairo was world's largest producer of velvet.

SEVERAL TYPES OF VELVET

Crushed Velvet

When the fabric is pressed down in different directions, crushed type of velvet is produced. It is also produced by twisting the fabric mechanically when it is wet. It is a good type of velvet, quite soft and ideal for children

Devore Velvet

Caustic solution produces such kind of velvet. This solution dissolves the part of velvet except for the area of fabric.

Embossed Velvet

To produce this pattern, a metal roller is used to heat-stamp the fabric. It is also a good type. Ladies love to wear it.

Hammered Velvet

It is somewhat like crushed velvet lustrous as well as dappled.

Panne Velvet

It's a new type of crushed velvet. It is produced by forcing the pile in a single direction. Heavy pressure is applied on it to make it softer.

Plain Velvet

It is simple, made of cotton and is used for many purposes apart from dresses and children outfits.

Silk Velvet It is also known as velvet type but it is more expensive than plain velvet. This type is usually shiner and softer than the cotton variety.

Viscose Velvet

It is also a kind of velvet which is more similar to silk velvet than cotton velvet

Chapter Seventeen

Fast Food: Healthy or Unhealthy

The craze for fast food is prevalent. Fast food outlets every here and there are mushrooming. They are favourite haunts for both youngsters and working couples. Do you ever think the food you eat at several food joints is actually nutritious for you?

The doctors say that the fast food, which is also known as junk food such as pizzas, chips, noodles, soft aerated drinks, ice cream, burgers, to some extent, is neither economical nor does it provide a balanced diet.

No doubt, these fast foods satisfy our taste and are available conveniently. They provide us instant gratification also but they are nonstop source of fats and cholesterol resulting the obesity and horrible diseases at later stage.

We need calories but these foods are empty of them. Even street foods such as tikkis, samosas, kachoris, panipuris, gol gappas etc. are also cooked in unhealthy conditions making them unhealthier than the same foods made at home.

Then, what should we do? Should we absolutely banish these foods from our diet and stick to conventional, boring, fat free diets to stay healthy? Or should we continue eating fast, junk food to relish the transitory satisfaction forgetting the long-term harm to our body. Do you know how you can make your fast food healthy? First, you know the effects of fast food on your body.

The Effects of Fast Food on Body

These foods are empty of nutrients and have very high fat contents. Fat contents cause hardening of coronary arteries which become the reason of heart ailments and stroke.

Scientifically, it has proved that sugar foods such as rasgula and gulab jamun, burfi etc. also lead to obesity, increase in cholesterol, high blood pressure and eventually cardiac problems such as angina.

These foods are high in carbohydrates the substance also leads to obesity inviting the series of ailments.

These foods contain monosodium glutamate and several other preservatives and additives which are also harmful to the body. In these food, high salt contents are used which give hypertension.

Ashwini Ahuja

Make Your Fast Food Healthy

Dr. Arun Makkar says that the more you eat fast food, the more leptin hormone, which is strongly related to weight and appetite; in your body releases more signals to brain increasing your eating impulse.

Don't let your brain to increase the impulse of excessive eating. But, it doesn't mean that you lose your heart and deprive yourself from enjoying the interesting food. Follow these guidelines while enjoying the food of your fancy.

1   Visit the fast food shop of your choice, drink fresh fruit juice, fat free sweetened milk or numbu jal (lemon water) in place of aerated drinks.

2   Enjoy your pizza but not binge on. Eat a smaller portion. Make sure, there are lots of vegetable and lettuces on its topping.

3   Never make fast food your staple diet.

4   Avoid ice cream. If necessary take milk shake or mango, banana shake etc.

5   If you are taking a burger, take it half and moreover, don't forget taking a plate of salad before it to reduce its intake.

6   Limit the portion of cheese, creamy potatoes and of macroni salads.

7   Never eat pizza base if it is empty of veggies.

8   If you like to relish non vegetarian, choose roasted or grilled kitchen.

Chapter Eighteen

Love Your Pizza, but Not Binge On

Most of us, men and women, love to relish yummy pizza as it is one of the most famous junk foods across the world which is also known as "the Queen" of the Mediterranean Diet.

Either you are at home or at workplace, pizza is everywhere to delight in your mood. But, most of us are also afraid of obesity only due to pizza. For some people, pizza is labeled as an unhealthy food. The question: Is it really an unhealthy food?

Consult Your Doctor

No doubt, most pizzas are high in saturated fat, salt and calories but if you are eating a balanced diet and having workout as well just about some forty-fifty minutes regularly, you needn't be worried a bit.

If you are overweight and don't have active lifestyle then you must check the quality of ingredients used in pizza preparation or consult the doctor necessarily before devouring pizza. High calories pizzas are not good for those persons who lack time for exercises.

Reducing the risk of Cancer

Excess of everything is bad. Renowned Nutritionist Ishi Khosla, Escort says; don't call pizza a junk food. It's undoubtedly a diet for health but if you binge on it you might invite obesity and several other ailments.

A report of researchers working at Mario Negri Institute for Pharmaceutical Research Centre, Milan says that eating pizza at least once a week regularly reduces the risk of developing oesophageal cancer by 59%, colon cancer by 26%; mouth cancer by 34%. It is also helpful in protecting against tumors and cardiovascular disaster.

Cook Pizza Expertly

According to study by the physicians of Harvard Medical School, men who consume tomatoes, tomato sauce or pizza more than twice a week reduce the risk factor of prostate cancer by thirty four percent as compared to those who didn't consume pizza food. Overall, pizza is healthy if it is prepared expertly, the experts claim.

The Food Chemists of Maryland University are of the view that different temperatures and cooking times determine the quality of baked pizza. Higher temperature and shorter time for pizza cooking is quite unsafe.

Dr. Ravindera Lavania says probably antioxidants can increase by as much as 80-85 percent if it is not properly cooked at moderate temperature, so cooking determines its healthy factor.

Quantity for Consumption

A single slice of pizza contains 250-500 calories. Moreover, the sodium level in an ordinary pizza is also very high- over 1,000 mg of sodium.

Dr. Ishi Khosla states that it is healthy if you don't eat too much of it. Dr. Pankaj Aneja, PGI Chandigarh says that just one or two slices are nutritious, five or six slices are definitely harmful. USA based dietician Ms. Diane Feasley also says that pizza consumption in moderation is alright.

There are nutrients associated with every food. One should not eliminate it from diet but practice moderation. She further suggests one must eat salad with pizza to practice balance and prevent oneself from consuming just pizza.

If one thinks being slim is one's target for health and for this, he lacks essential nutrients he might give harm to every part of his body. Eating smaller portions of pizza is certainly beneficial.

Pizza: A Source of Lycopene

Ashwini Ahuja

Tomato or tomato products especially sauce- which is a source of lycopene is used in pizza. It is better absorbed when pizza is cooked with fat such as oil and cheese. While preparing pizza, process of tomatoes lycopene increases. Lycopene in processed tomato is four times higher than in fresh tomatoes unlike most vegetables where nutritional contents reduce with its cooking. Physicians say that the antioxidant effects of lycopene- the most prevalent caroteniod in human blood plasma- are much strong.

Lycopene protects the human body against the damaging effects of free radicals which are linked to cancer and cardiovascular and some chronic diseases.

Dr. Amit Sachdeva suggests that one should consume at least 6 mg of lycopene regularly which reduces the risk of prostate cancer. He further says that tomatoes and tomato products- pasteurised tomato juices, sauce, soups are best sources of lycopene.

Dr. Amit further advises one should eat pizzas which are cooked in olive oil. Just the sprinkling of cheese is enough for healthy and moderate pizza.

Dr. Vijay Thakker of "Thakker Hospital" opines pizza is quite healthy because fresh tomatoes and olive oil (which are generally used in pizza) really work better. This combination enhances lycopene absorption. Lycopene is fat soluble and oil helps absorption. He further adds, if one ingests just 12 mg (in the case of women, 6.5 mg) of tomato products regularly, the risk of lung cancer can also be reduced provided one is non-smoker.

Home Based Pizza Is Better

Housewife Mamta Jain of Hanumangarh says, in most Indian families, pizza is greatly loved but pizza stuff sold in market is high in fat, sodium and calories which lead to being overweight and obese.

No doubt, some renowned pizza houses make natural pizzas specifically counting the calories but in general, pizzas sold on unspecified shops are unhealthiest things. She adds that even some leading shops don't use whole wheat crusts so if you are able to prepare pizza at home that is much better. If not, don't eat more than one slice of pizza at restaurant. Eat healthy green salad first to balance your pizza diet. Be alert; don't end up eating more than half of the pizza.

Mamta further says that while making pizza at home; make it with a thin crust and put only a little cheese and log of veggies on it. One can also use quality ingredients.

The best point is: homemade pizza will never ooze as much oil as restaurant pizza does. Sushma Mukherjee, a teacher in Haridwar, says it is hundred percent true, moderate pizzas can help all those who are striving to lose weight.

How Pizza is helpful in losing weight

Ashwini Ahuja

Dr. Rishu Makkar, MD opines, undoubtedly, pizza can help one who wants to lose weight. One must be careful regarding the portion and the calories in that piece. If one eats negative calorie foods with pizza, it can benefit one's health. If you opt for negative calorie veggies and fruits such as spinach, carrot, cucumber, lettuce, asparagus, zucchini, orange, watermelon, pineapple, cantaloupe and eggplant etc. you can definitely lose your weight. These are such foods which burn more calories when they are eaten than they actually consist of.

Origin of Pizza

Sandeep Jhinja, lecturer in History says- "pizza" is an old Italian word which means- "a point". Its other name is "pizzicare" which means- "to pinch" or "to pluck". Needless to mention, pizza- a baked pie originates from Italy.

No doubt, it must have been invented by the Greeks or Romans and they knew the secrets of blending flour with water and heating it on stone. Since the Stone Age, pizza has been an essential part of Italian diet. In old times, pizza was baked beneath of stones of the fire. The American noticed pizza in 1950s.

History of Pizza

Pizza dates back to the neolithic age. Its history is as old as bread. The people of Ancient Greek added some ingredients- herbs, onion and garlic to bread (also called it Plakous) to make the pizza more palatable. The soldiers of "Darius- the Great"- the Persian King baked bread and covered it with dates and cheese. It was the 18th century when a group of people in Naples also used to add tomato to yeast based flat bread.

Later, the same food pie was called pizza. Thanks to its tempting taste, the dish earned popularity in a short period. It became an attraction for the tourists to Naples. Even vendors and open-air stands began to sell pizzas to common folks.

Antica Pizzeria Port'Alba was known as the first of all pizzerias in Naples which in 1830 was expanded to pizza restaurant but back in 1738, it had started its preparation for peddlers. A French writer and food expert Alexandre Dumas in his book writes, during winter season, pizza was considered the only food for humble people.

Pizza in USA

In USA, pizza gave its bang in 19th century. It was most popular in Italian immigrants in USA so preferably, it was sold in San Francisco, Chicago, New York City and Philadelphia where the Italian immigrants, in those days, were hugely populated.

Before 1940, its consumption remained limited to Italian immigrants. After the World War II, soldiers who were looking for good food discovered the pizzeria and tasted the good stuff of pizza.

Ashwini Ahuja

Later, pizza reached to India and South Asian countries. The pizza base in Naples was soft and pliable. In Rome, foodies love thin and crispy base. In Italy, pizza is baked in rectangular tray. In old times, tomatoes in pizzas were not as profusely used as they are used today.

How to Make your Pizza Healthy

1. Always use a thin crust. Use only wheat flour. Pre-made whole wheat pizza crust can also be purchased from the market.
2. Give it delectable taste by using basil, garlic powder and oregano.
3. Use only olive oil. It reduces bad cholesterol.
4. Always use tomato based sauce. Tomatoes are an excellent source of vitamins A and C
5. Low fat cheese which is an excellent source of calcium is good for health in pizza.
6. Veggie topping is good; if you are meat lover, use the leanest topping but the choice of onions, tomatoes, spinach, peppers, mushrooms and broccoli can make the pizza a different stuff.
7. Add no sweet to your dough.
8. Never use greasy processed meats.

Techniques for Moderate Pizza

In view of fitness and nutritious point, pizza should be baked in wood-fired oven. It must not be baked more than at 485°C. Baking time should be not more than one to three minutes. Its base must be hand-kneaded. In diameter, it must not be exceeded 35 centimeters. Its centre point should be quite thick and stuffy.

Facts about Pizza

February 9 is known as an International Pizza Day

Guinness Book of World Records shows the largest ever 100 feet and 1 inch pizza was prepared and eaten in Havana

Pizza is most popular in America, Canada and India. In America 23 pounds of pizza is eaten per person per year.

Celebrities Jerry Colonna, Jimmy Durante, Frank Sinatra and baseball celebrity Joe DiMaggio ate pizza ravenously.

Dean Martin, a famous singer had sung a song- *When the moon hits your eye like a big pizza pie, that a more-* on the significance and beauty of pizza.

Chapter Nineteen

Internet Banking

Internet banking is the need of recent times. Almost all the banks of the private sector as well the public sector offers the facility of internet banking to their customers. Due to the plethora of safety measures and RBI guidelines, internet banking today is quite safe provided you must have to be cautious while you enjoy the facility at your home or at your office.

Generally, customers opt for this service for transaction and check their balance in their account. If you are enrolled for internet banking, you can also avail of a number of other value-added services apart from transaction and checking the balance in your account.

Funds transfer Facility It is the best one facility, the mainstream banks provide to their customers. Through this facility, the customers can transfer their funds to the other accounts within the same branch or any other branch of the same bank in other cities of India. The second type: the facility allows the internet banking customers to transfer funds electronically to accounts in others banks within India.

For fund transfer, there are two types of service available. They are known as NEFT (National Electronic Fund Transfer) and RTGS (Real Times Gross Settlement)

In NEFT service, there is no minimum limit on the amount of money that can be transferred from 8 a.m to 4 p.m all days except for Saturday. On Saturday, the service is available for half day by 11.30 a.m. The maximum limit through NEFT is varied from five lakhs to more.

Through NEFT, funds are sent to RBI within three hours of the transaction but the credit of the payment depends on the time taken by the beneficiary bank to process the payment. On the other hand, The RTGS system is the fastest possible inter bank money transfer facility.

The fund through this system is transferred from one bank to another on a real time and on gross settlement basis. The minimum limit on the amount of money that can be transferred through RTGS is one lakh and maximum is five lakh or more depend on the facilities provided by the banks.

Facility of the Demand Draft

If you want to get demand drafts, you need not visit the bank and fill the form for it. Through internet banking, this facility is also available. At the website of the bank, first of all, you have to choose the account from which the amount for the demand draft has to be debited. Simply enter the amount and the name of the beneficiary and then the name of the branch at which the draft is payable.

After that, banks provide two types of facilities, either you collect the demand draft in person or ask the bank authority to send it to you through courier. But for confirmation, you need to generate the counter foil and take the print-out.

In public sector banks, demand drafts up to the value of 10,000 are issued without charging any commission. For demand drafts up to the value of one lakh, commission just Rs: 50 and the demand draft up to the value of 5 lakhs, the commission Rs: 100 is charged.

Pay Your Bills Online Facility

It is boon for all customers. They can pay their all types of bills- electricity, insurance, telephone, etc. online by using this facility from your home or office. You need not to go to electricity or LIC office and stand in a queue there. By paying online, you can save your precious time, energy and paper. How you have to use this facility.

Simple, just visit your bank website, click the links as per your requirements. And your all bills will be paid within minutes and amount will get deducted from your account.

After paying the bills, the bank will also send you an SMS or email alert for confirmation and let you know the amount has been debited from your account. After having paid the bill, the transaction number will appear on the screen. You can save it for your future reference. You bills can also be paid automatically whenever they are due if you set the instructions on your computer.

Tax Deduction Facility

You can pay your tax thorough online. Also, this facility will allow you to generate the details of tax deducted from your account during the previous financial year. Projected TDS for the current financial year can also be generated within 30 minutes.

It can also help you to your future tax planning. You can print the TDS details and get the document signed by the concerned bank official. It will then act as a TDS certificate that you can submit to the income tax department.

Safety Measures

By using these facilities, you must be aware of the safety of your account. Undoubtedly banks provide full security but you must be aware on your part for safe internet banking. Be aware regarding the use of predictable password. Never write the password at insecure place where the other can access it. Don't forget change the password every three months and don't choose your date of birth, car number or telephone or mobile number as your password.

The longer the password, the better it is. Don't forget to sign off your account after its use. Make transaction on your computer. If you use other computer, don't forget to log off completely and close the page finally. If someone contacts you through email or telephone and claims to be the representative of bank, don't give them any information regarding your account. Contact the bank to verify the request.

Chapter Twenty

DESIGNER JEWELLERY

Every woman and girl loves to look extremely beautiful, stylish and classy. Other than trendy, cool and crazy apparels and footwear, she also loves to wear designer jewellery to make her appearance more attractive, elegantly great and above all, pleasing to all eyes.

Nisha Verma, a jeweller says that generally, for ladies, jewellery is a unique form of distinctive style statement and they happily spend considerable money on ornaments as they believe that their jewels will show the people how well-off and prosperous the wearer ladies are.

Market trends show that the fashion of designer jewellery is on the up and in the coming years, it is bound to shoot up spectacularly both in domestic and international markets. At present, designer jewellery ornaments are available only in selected showrooms of big cities but the in the coming days, such jewellery will hit the markets of small cities and towns.

Nisha Verma says that on account of new millennium ladies' interest for designer jewellery, showroom owners and jewellery marking executives are quite confident that the sale would definitely shoot up as they have geared up all for proper marketing and distribution system. Needless to say that Indian designer jewellery has carved a niche for itself in Europe, America, Australia and Gulf countries, Nisha concludes.

JEWELLERY CONVEYS STYLE AND TASTE

Since ages, jewellery has been woman's first obsessive love. Every woman has the passion for pretty jewellery. She loves to wear ornaments tastefully. Some like it as it makes them feel good when they wear it. Nisha Verma says that some ladies perhaps wear the jewellery to brag their social status also. While some others wear it simply as it looks pretty.

At present, the trend has certainly changed. Today, women generally love to wear DJ (designer jewellery) in preference to conventional jewellery because such ornaments convey one's style and taste. As for the designer jewellery, one can enjoy wearing it for a very reasonable and affordable price.

Such jewellery is available on several jewellery houses. Expensive materials such as gold, diamond and real precious stones are not used in such jewellery in view of the risk factor of pillaging or attack on ladies.

Moreover, such innovative jewellery makes the ladies' looks more eye-catching. In such jewellery, innovative designs are made with Plastic cut stones.

Nisha Verma reminds that similar kind of jewellery had become popular during Victorian era and its popularity still has not diminished rather it has developed itself with innovation in its designs.

NRI ladies also prefer such jewellery as it is worn on all occasions and go well with any kind of costume either formal or casual.

Moreover, it is light wear and elegant. Not only the ordinary ladies but the celebrities like Julia Robert, Britney Spears and Bollywood princesses also love to wear designer jewellery.

STYLE IN GOLD

Ashwini Ahuja

Undoubtedly, gold jewellery is good for all seasons. It is available in different designs in several jewellery showrooms along with diamond studded ornaments. "Style in gold" is a new buzz word to cater the needs and choices of the gold-lover customers.

Jewellery connoisseurs say that gold is beautiful, malleable, attractive and non reactive with other elements, it doesn't discolor; so it never goes out of fashion. Women's love for gold is hundred percent pure and true. Moreover, jewellers can give gold into any shape and contour including tiny strands that can be used for gold necklace jewellery. Unquestionably, gold necklace jewellery is in vogue. It is supreme, matchless and perfect and moreover it is loved by one and all.

Above all, for most Indian women, gold is still the safest investment and it also delights their lure for traditional jewellery. So, a number of rich and fashionable young women also buy gold jewellery in addition to get her hands on designer jewellery.

THE BEAUTY OF PURE GOLD

If you are planning to give orders for gold necklace jewellery, be sure in choosing the right gold. Jewellers classify gold into four categories- 24 karat, 18 karat, 14 karat and 10 karat.

24 karat is considered as a pure gold while 18 karat contains 18 parts of gold and 6 parts of other metals.

Other metals make 18 karat 75 percent pure. So, right gold is 24 karat. It is 99.9 percent pure. It is quite soft and it is practical to wear.

Remember that a negligible mixture of other metal in gold is good for its durability, so when you place order for jewellery, prefer to mix the bare minimum fraction of other metal for its durability.

When gold is mixed with other metals in more than 5-6 percent, it changes colour after some time and lose its luster. If you are interested to wear white gold to make your looks more charming and charismatic, ask the jewellers to mix nickel or palladium in 24 karat pure gold.

HISTORY BECKONS

If we look back the history of jewellery, it was worn by both men and women thousands of years back. Archaeological excavations show that people also wore some form of primitive jewellery before they started to live in houses.

When they started to live in their own houses, they started to wear other types of ornaments. These types at present are known as antique jewellery. Jewellery connoisseurs say that all the jewellery that is pre-owned is considered as antique jewellery.

This type of jewellery is unique and very different in its designs and makings. Everybody loves to have such jewellery at least one piece of it. Now-a-days, jewellery designers also try to give the antique looks to its latest jewellery to attract the lady customers.

JEWELLERY FOR ALL FESTIVALS

In country like India, fashion and trends change as fast as none even can imagine. One item hits the market one moment before another product steals the spotlight in just a short span of time.

Ashwini Ahuja

Today, the trend of innovative design jewellery has emerged in both wholesale and retail jewellery markets. Needless to say that today, whole sale jewellery is not just about selling the ornaments in bulk. Wholesalers also sell their products in retails to increase their sale.

During festivals, they attract the customers announcing several beneficial schemes for them. With the changed time, ladies love to wear theme jewellery on festival seasons that is available with wholesale traders as well as on retail showrooms or stores.

During Diwali days, Ganesha pendants, earring in the shape of diyas (earthen pot) and jewellery with 3-D images of Goddess Luxmi are very popular. Jewellers don't miss any opportunity to swell their sale whether it is an auspicious occasion of Ganesh Chaturthi, Raksha Bandhan, Holi or Mother Day.

On the special day of Valentine, heart shaped pendants are sold in myriad. Nisha Verma says that really the time has now incredibly changed. At present, gold now comes in myriad colours ranging from rose, white, red, pink to green and purple. Such recipe of different colours reflects the mood of Holi festival.

Mamta Jain, a housewife says that today the time has miraculously changed. The new millennium ladies want customized jewellery. It should be unique, elegant and fashionable, they desire. Its designs should speak for themselves and moreover the jewellery should tone with the mood of every occasion.

Now-a-days, most emerging designers have created their individual styles to tap the jewellery market. They are targeting both festivals and special occasions by featuring different items including coral, turquoise, agates as well as rose quartz etc. Earlier, these items were available from rock and gem wholesaler or big suppliers etc. but today, the scenario has totally changed.

SILVER JEWELLERY FOR ALL SEASONS

Designer silver jewellery is also in vogue. Women love to wear it on special occasions. It is versatile and suited for all seasons.

Mamta Jain says that designer silver jewellery is so unique that one may have the feelings of warmness by wearing an amber colour stones-studded glowing pair of silver earring even in the chilly cold. In summer, a silver ankle chain or glittering necklace can add the charm of summer dress.

In silver jewellery, one may discover much more varieties of styles and designs suited for all occasions from wedding to routine office work. Ladies love to wear plains designs for home or office as they are considered ideals.

You can get off wearing anything with unique silver jewellery. Heavy chunky ornaments through the winter months are ideal as they look identical with heavy clothing. If it is summer, you may wear light, petite jewellery.

Ashwini Ahuja

Nisha Verma suggests that whether silver jewellery is not so precious but you must verify before buying the silver jewellery whether the seller is upright and trustworthy. If he is not, don't buy jewellery from him. Examine his business details. Read terms and conditions of that company. If the terms and conditions provide good service to the customers and the company or showroom is genuine and is dedicated for good services, then you must visit the showroom for shopping.

PEARLS FOR ALL SEASONS

Anshu Bala, a jewellery connoisseur opines that designer pearl jewellery is matchless, amazing and in vogue as well. It is no less than gold, silver or trendy jewels. The best point in wearing pearls jewellery is that it doesn't ruin in rainy season.

One can enjoyably drench herself in rainy seasons wearing peals sets because it is sure that they will not get ruined or stained. Silver and gold jewelry may lose its shine after your several showers in rain.
If you love to wear pearls then no matter what season, pearls are fine in every season. They are smooth, glossy and in round shape.

They are produced inside the shell of oyster. In ancient Rome and Egypt, people regarded them as the best symbol of power, wealth and prosperity.

Pearls are of several colours but generally white colour pearls are used for ornaments or trendy jewellery. Unlike several other gem stones, they don't require any particular season for its adornment. Apart from jewellery, pearls are used in making gift sets. In winter, some ladies love to titivate pearls on sweaters or hand bags to bragger their richness.

CRAZE FOR DIAMONDS

Gone are the days when the diamonds were considered for only affluent and rich people. Today, there are almost fourteen thousand categories of diamonds which are available in the market, so, in the present time, diamond for every budget is available in the market. Like gold, diamond is also considered a sound long term investment.

Mrs. Reema Thatai, sale advisor of diamond jewellery suggests that ladies should be aware while buying diamond jewellery. There are several chances of frauds in diamond industry if you are not alert in buying diamonds. Two diamonds of the same size may differ widely in quality.

She suggests that while buying jewellery, one should understand the cut, colour, clarity and carat weight of the diamond. A better cut gives more brilliance. Brilliant cut in the world has 57 facets. Brilliant cut diamonds come in a range of shapes. Clarity also much matters, Reema concludes.

BEWARE OF FRAUDS

Ashwini Ahuja

Reema Thatai next says that some ladies wear particular special jewellery or white gold necklaces as a symbol of good fortune. For them, white gold jewellery must have a powerful spiritual meaning but you should not think that all white gold jewellery is really good, fine and original. Over the past years, jewellery markets have flooded with duplicate and bogus jewellery pieces.

Online shopping sites such as eBay.com is displaying jewellery such as rings, earrings and necklaces that look almost identical to one that cost 2-3 lakhs. They are actually on sale for just Rs: 500-600. So, always beware of such frauds and deceitful practices.

LADIES IN GENERAL SAY

1. Wearing jewellery is a form of human expression of wealth and personality
2. They wish to cheer themselves up so; they wear unique jewellery and ornaments.
3. Jewellery enhances the beauty of their dress and outfits.
4. If you want to outshine in any night party or festival, have a collection of both designer vintage and antique jewellery.
5. They wear jewellery that is in sync with the clothes they wear.
6. Jewellery that has designs like flower petals are loved by both girls and ladies

Chapter Twenty One

Chuck Out Body Odour

Ashwini Ahuja

Despite taking several precautions, in summer, sometimes, we experience an awkward situation because of the unbearable & unpleasant sweat odour our body emanates. We try to stay clean and odourless but it is not always possible if we don't remain alert.

Moreover, we have to spend long hours outdoors under the scorching sun and our body often perspires. No doubt, sweat is a protective liquid secreted by sweat glands. It actually cools us in the heat but sometimes it smells unpleasantly and we feel embarrassed in the good company of our colleagues or friends.

Sweat Is Good For Body

Dr. Pankaj Aneja PGI, Chandigarh says actually, sweat is natural and good for the body. Sweat itself is odourless. The bacterial flora on the surface of the skin is the cause of odour. It acts upon the sweat and releases odour, sometimes odour becomes unbearable.

Dr. Arun Makkar, MD clarifies that every person has different flora so the smell in every person is quite different, even some bodies don't smell either. Also, some types of bacteria are not in our control system, Dr. Makkar opines, but we can get rid of body odour by following some methods which definitely let the sweat cool without annoying odour.

Opt For Right Deodorant

Dr. Arun Makkar suggests that we should always opt for right deodorant. There are two types. First type is anti-perspirant which is quite harmful as this type blocks the sweat. It is not a good sign for the health of the body and the mind. The second type is for masking the odour. It is quite good but its regular use is risky for health.

For ladies & girls, natural fruit deodorants are satisfactory as they smell good and at the same time, they are not very strong scented. Be ensured you are not using alcohol based deodorants. They can blacken your underarms instead.

In later stage, it can also cause sun allergies and other skin problems. Dr. Amit Sachdeva of IGMC Shimla says that plant derived fragrant oils in the deodorant which is in every type of products can cause pigmentation also.

He further suggests if you are going for a party or job interview, you can apply deodorant but not regularly. We should use talc power every morning after a bath because it is absolutely harmless. It cools the body and absorbs sweat and unwanted dampness.

No Repeated Bath Daily

Ashwini Ahuja

Bath is good for health. It refreshes and rejuvenates our body but Dr. Shweta Parnami, a dermatologist opines that you should never shower repeatedly as it can reduce the bacteria on your skin and remove the oily layer off the skin consequently making it chapped & dry.

Chapped skin is most likely exposed to cuts and wounds inviting bacteria to stay there.

Dr. Shweta further says, in summer season, if you want to bathe twice or thrice, you must not use soap repeatedly. At the time of bath, you must wash your armpits adequately, she advises.

To remove the body smell, one can alternatively use scented shower gel plus anti-bacterial soap or moisture based cleanser. Take bath everyday—if possible but not repeatedly. Dry yourself well after a bath. Dry your armpits, toes etc. because the bacteria and fungi thrive in moist environments. They cause bad odour.

Wear Loose Cotton Outfits

Cotton clothes relax our body and let the breeze touch our inner body parts. They help us in sweat evaporate and doesn't cause skin inflammation or dermatitis so always wear roomy and airy outfits. Never wear tight clothes.

In tight clothes, you can let the sweat collect in a spot which creates body odour. Forget the synthetic clothes especially in summer season that are purely made of nylon and polyester. Shave your armpit hair from time to time, if not possible regularly, do it at least twice or thrice a week; it will remain the area clear of bacteria.

And when you came back home from office or the working place, change your outfits promptly. Don't ever wear the same clothes for office next day.

Choose Leather Footwear

Leather footwear is anti odour. Wear it while going to party or working place. Maintain two or more pairs of footwear. Try not to wear the same pair for two or more days in a row. Synthetic footwear and socks are not good choice for summer season. Wear cotton socks preferably. They absorb sweat better than synthetic material. Change socks and undergarments everyday. Give your feet enough air. When you are at home, keep your feet bare. Don't wear socks when you are at home for rest.

Drink Water Abundantly

Start your morning with sufficient drinking water. The more your drink water, the more you cool down your body and feel fresh the all day. Also, water helps the body flush out toxins resulting dying away the body's bad odour.

Dr. Anju Setia advises that one must drink at least 10-15 glasses of water daily apart from several nutritious liquids viz. juice, lemonade, coconut water, sharbat, lassi and water based seasonal fruits such as watermelon and muskmelon etc. in summer to discourage dehydration.

Ashwini Ahuja

Dr. Arun Makkar says that it is better if you keep yourself hydrated and detoxified making sure your system of throwing out waste products otherwise the wastes will find outlet through unbearable, bad smelly sweat.

Keep Your Bacteria in Check

Another way to keep your bacteria in check is vinegar-water mixture. It is an easy method which can be applied easily at home.

Dr. Amit Sachdeva says that vinegar is acetic acid which discourages bacteria from multiplying. He also advises the method of application. Apply this mixture to your skin with cotton. This way, one can remove the bacteria on skin.

He further says that diabetes and obesity can also invite smelly sweating, so check up on your weight and avoid junk food.

No Peppery Food

Dr. Ravindra Lavania says that junk and spicy or peppery food is also the cause of the body odour. Minimize to eat junk and spicy food. Eat a lot of home made food, rice, roti, salad and veggies. The food containing caffeine like tea, coffee & chocolate should be taken in a smaller amount. The earlier you stop having such food the faster you stop sweat smelling.

Dr. Lavania further says that food like onion and garlic could affect the smell of the sweat also. Also eat less the foods such as red meat that trigger sweating and body odour in you.

Control Your Stress

Dr. Amit Sachdeva says that stress is also one of the causes of unpleasant odour in our bodies. We can try to get rid of it by doing light exercises. Going to gym twice or thrice a week can also be a good option to eradicate the stress.

Moreover, if you are quiet hesitant in visiting gym, meditation or yoga at home also can help you in controlling the stress.

Why Body Smells Unpleasantly

In our skin, we have two types of sweat glands-Eccrine Glands and Apocrine Glands. Eccrine Glands cover the most parts of our body surface. Apocrine Glands covers the area where there are abundance of hair growth in our body such as armpits, scalp & groin etc.

When the temperature of the body rises, the sweat brain signals the Eccrine Glands to release sweat appears on the surface of skin. This sweat cools the body and maintains its temperature.

Apocrine glands release fatty sweat, not on the surface of the skin but into the small tubes of the glands. Then, the fatty sweat is pushed out onto the surface of the skin where bacteria start the process of sweating causing unpleasant body odour. We can't smell ourselves.

Only others can tell us if our bodies release foul odour. Sweat is composed mainly of water and salt plus containing small amounts of other electrolytes-substances which help in regulating the balance of fluid in the body.

Ashwini Ahuja